Obesity Mana

Louis J. Aronne • Rekha B. Kumar
Editors

Obesity Management

A Clinical Casebook

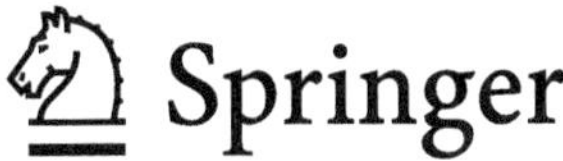

Editors
Louis J. Aronne
NewYork–Presbyterian Hospital
Weill Cornell Medical College
New York, NY
USA

Rekha B. Kumar
NewYork–Presbyterian Hospital
Weill Cornell Medical College
New York, NY
USA

ISBN 978-3-030-01038-6 ISBN 978-3-030-01039-3 (eBook)
https://doi.org/10.1007/978-3-030-01039-3

Library of Congress Control Number: 2018965172

This Springer imprint is published by the registered company Springer Nature Switzerland AG
The registered company address is: Gewerbestrasse 11, 6330 Cham, Switzerland

Preface

As the prevalence of global obesity reaches pandemic proportions, it is our responsibility as physicians to learn current and effective interventions, give patients treatment options, and interact with patients with obesity in a compassionate manner. Despite our awareness of the increase in obesity prevalence and the known costs incurred due to complications of this disease, most physicians do not feel well-trained in treating patients with obesity or giving nutritional advice. A great advance in this area has been the creation of the American Board of Obesity Medicine (ABOM), which has now credentialed more than 2000 physicians in obesity medicine through a certification exam. This has led to a critical mass of physicians who have knowledge of the disease state and have shown competence in their understanding through passing the exam. Despite that, we are lacking in clinical training programs and practical educational tools on specific clinical scenarios that the obesity medicine physician may encounter.

In this clinical casebook, we asked obesity medicine providers at the Comprehensive Weight Control Center at Weill Cornell Medical College to help compile prototypical cases we see in our practice, which is dedicated to the state-of-the-art obesity treatment. Each chapter begins with a clinical scenario that depicts a patient with medically complicated obesity and then proceeds through assessment and diagnosis as well as options for a treatment plan. The cases culminate with a patient outcome and a summary of clinical pearls and pitfalls relevant to each patient scenario. We hope this clinical casebook can be a practical tool for educating physicians in the clinical care of patients with obesity.

New York, NY, USA Rekha B. Kumar, MD, DABOM
New York, NY, USA Louis J. Aronne, MD, DABOM

Conflict of Interest

Dr. Aronne reports receiving consulting fees from and/serving on advisory boards for Jamieson Laboratories, Pfizer, Novo Nordisk, Eisai, GI Dynamics, Real Appeal, Janssen, UnitedHealth Group Ventures, and Gelesis, receiving research funding from Aspire Bariatrics, Eisai, and AstraZeneca, having an equity interest in BMIQ, Zafgen, Gelesis, MYOS, and Jamieson Laboratories, and serving on a board of directors for MYOS, BMIQ, and Jamieson Laboratories. He is a consultant to Janssen Pharmaceuticals and Sanofi.

Dr. Rekha Kumar serves as the Medical Director of the American Board of Obesity Medicine. She reports serving as a speaker for Novo Nordisk and Janssen Pharmaceuticals, having equity interests in Vivus, Zafgen, and Myos Corporation.

New York, NY, USA — Rekha B. Kumar
New York, NY, USA — Louis J. Aronne

Contents

Contributors

Caroline A. Andrew, MD Hospital for Special Surgery, New York, NY, USA

Ana B. Emiliano, MD, DABOM The Rockefeller University, Clinician at the Comprehensive Weight Control Center, Weill Cornell Medical Center, New York, NY, USA

Janet Feinstein, MSRD Comprehensive Weight Control Center, Division of Endocrinology, Diabetes and Metabolism, Weill Cornell Medical College, New York, NY, USA

Leon I. Igel, MD, DABOM Comprehensive Weight Control Center, Division of Endocrinology, Diabetes and Metabolism, Weill Cornell Medical College, New York, NY, USA

Rekha B. Kumar, MD, DABOM Comprehensive Weight Control Center, Division of Endocrinology, Diabetes and Metabolism, Weill Cornell Medical College, New York, NY, USA

Rachel Lustgarten, RDN Comprehensive Weight Control Center, Division of Endocrinology, Diabetes and Metabolism, Weill Cornell Medical College, New York, NY, USA

Lindsay Mandel, BA Weill Cornell Medical College, New York, NY, USA

Katherine H. Saunders, MD, DABOM Comprehensive Weight Control Center, Division of Endocrinology, Diabetes and Metabolism, Weill Cornell Medical College, New York, NY, USA

Alpana Shukla, MD Comprehensive Weight Control Center, Division of Endocrinology, Diabetes and Metabolism, Weill Cornell Medical College, New York, NY, USA

Beverly G. Tchang, MD Comprehensive Weight Control Center, Division of Endocrinology, Diabetes and Metabolism, Weill Cornell Medical College, New York, NY, USA

Devika Umashanker, MD, DABOM Department of Bariatric Surgery, Hartford Hospital, Hartford, CT, USA

Part I
Metabolic Syndrome

Chapter 1
Identifying and Treating the Metabolic Syndrome

Caroline A. Andrew

Case Presentation

A 45-year-old male presents to an obesity medicine specialist for evaluation. His body mass index (BMI) is 40 kg/m^2. His past medical history is significant for hypertension (HTN) and dyslipidemia. Medications include hydrochlorothiazide, losartan, rosuvastatin, and a daily aspirin. Blood pressure has been difficult to control despite his medications, and his cardiologist is considering adding a third agent. Family history is notable for both parents with obesity and HTN; his father had bariatric surgery. One of his sisters is overweight and has type 2 diabetes. He works as the manager of a construction company and is on his feet most of the day. He denies any use of tobacco and drinks one to two beers every night. His typical diet consists of a breakfast of eggs and toast, and then he will typically eat out for lunch and dinner, often stopping for dinner at fast-food restaurants on his way home.

On review of systems, he denies having any chest pain, shortness of breath, palpitations, or lower extremity edema.

C. A. Andrew (✉)
Hospital for Special Surgery, New York, NY, USA
e-mail: andrewca@hss.edu

L. J. Aronne, R. B. Kumar (eds.), *Obesity Management*,
https://doi.org/10.1007/978-3-030-01039-3_1

His exam is notable for a blood pressure of 140/90 mmHg and heart rate of 78 bpm. His waist circumference is 43 in. Recent fasting labs are remarkable for glucose 103 mg/dL, low-density lipoprotein cholesterol (LDL-C) 112 mg/dL, high-density lipoprotein cholesterol (HDL-C) 38 mg/dL, and triglycerides 170 mg/dL.

Assessment and Diagnosis

This patient presents with class III obesity (BMI > 40 kg/m^2) and the metabolic syndrome. Body mass index (BMI) is used as a screening tool for overweight and obesity, by assessing a person's weight in relation to height. A BMI of 18.5–24.9 is considered normal. A BMI of 25.0–29.9 is overweight, and class I obesity is defined by BMI 30–34.9, class II BMI 35–39.9, and class III BMI of 40 or higher [1]. The 2013 American Heart Association/American College of Cardiology/The Obesity Society (AHA/ACC/TOS) guideline for the management of overweight and obesity in adults recommends that patients be screened at least annually by measuring height and weight and calculating BMI. Patients who fall in the overweight or obese range are at risk for cardiovascular disease (CVD), and those who have BMI >30 are at elevated mortality risk from all causes [2]. BMI is an excellent screening tool, but it is also important to identify patients who have a BMI within the normal range, but who present with comorbidities commonly associated with obesity, such as type 2 diabetes or the metabolic syndrome. The National Institute for Health and Clinical Excellence (NICE) guidelines support the use of lower BMI thresholds in the Asian populations (23 kg/m^2 for increased risk and 27.5 kg/m^2 for high risk) for further evaluation and treatment [3]. The AHA/ACC/TOS guideline also recommends the inclusion of waist circumference measurement in the evaluation of a patient [2]. Evidence demonstrates that cardiovascular risk increases with increased waist circumference, although there is a lack of strong evidence supporting the use of specific waist circumference cutoff points as markers for increased risk. Until further evidence is available, the guidelines recommend the continuing use of the cutoff points included in the National Institutes of Health/National Heart, Lung, and Blood Institute (NIH/NHLBI) or World Health Organization/International Diabetes Foundation (WHO/IDF) guidelines, >40 in. in men and >35 in. in women, to identify patients at increased risk for CVD [4]. The IDF provides different cutoffs of waist circumference based on ethnicity [5].

BMI and measurement of waist circumference provide easy and accessible methods of measuring and screening; however, the medical assessment of a patient with obesity requires a comprehensive history and physical examination in order to fully assess for disease risk factors. With a history of HTN and dyslipidemia, as well as an elevated waist circumference, this patient shows a high likelihood of having the metabolic syndrome. The metabolic syndrome is a condition defined by a constellation of risk factors for cardiovascular disease and/or type 2 diabetes. The American Heart Association (AHA) and NHLBI define the metabolic syndrome as having any three of the following criteria: elevated waist circumference (>40 in. in men, >35 in. in women), elevated triglycerides (>150 mg/dL or on treatment), reduced HDL-C (<40 mg/dL in men <50 mg/dL in women or on treatment), elevated blood pressure (>130 mm Hg systolic blood pressure or >85 mm Hg diastolic blood pressure or on treatment), and elevated fasting glucose (>100 mg/dL or on treatment). This patient meets all of the criteria for the metabolic syndrome [1].

Risk factors for the metabolic syndrome include obesity, specifically abdominal obesity, and insulin resistance [6, 7]. In the National Health and Nutrition Examination Survey III (NHANES III), the metabolic syndrome was present in 5% of those subjects with normal weight, 22% of those who were overweight, and 60% of subjects with obesity [8]. In the Framingham Heart Study, an increase in weight of 2.25 kg or more over 16 years was associated with a 21–45% increase in the risk of developing the metabolic syndrome [9]. In addition to obesity, other factors associated with increased risk of developing the metabolic syndrome include postmenopausal status, smoking, high carbohydrate diet, and limited physical activity.

Soft drink and sugar-sweetened beverage intake has also been associated with increased risk [9–11]. Medications, including antipsychotics, have been shown to increase risk. Finally, individuals with a family history of metabolic syndrome are at increased risk; genetic factors are thought to have a strong role in the development of the condition [12–14]. This patient's strong family history of obesity, HTN, and diabetes explains some of his own risk for developing the condition.

Management

Treatment of the metabolic syndrome focuses on modifiable risk reduction, including counseling regarding lifestyle changes to address obesity, physical inactivity, and diet. Drug therapy can also be considered to manage elevated LDL-C, blood pressure, and glucose [1].

First, this patient can be counseled about the importance of weight loss. Even modest weight loss of 3–5% is likely to be clinically significant and can reduce his level of triglycerides and fasting blood glucose and decrease his risk of developing type 2 diabetes [2]. If he can lose weight, he may see an improvement in his HTN, a decrease in LDL-C, and an increase in HDL-C and may be able to discontinue some of the medications he is currently taking to control his blood pressure and high cholesterol levels [2].

There are a variety of diets that can be offered to this patient. The AHA/ACC/TOS guideline for weight loss recommends either 1200–1500 kcal/day for women and 1500–1800 kcal/day for men (although these values should be adjusted for patient's body weight) or a 500 kcal/day–750 kcal/day energy-deficit or an evidence-based diet that restricts certain food types, thereby providing an energy-deficit [2].

The AHA/NHLBI have specific guidelines for the treatment of the metabolic syndrome. A goal weight reduction of 7–10% during the first year of treatment is recommended. For physical activity, individuals should aim for at least 30 min of continuous or intermittent moderate-intensity physical activity, at least 5 days per week. Resistance training should also be incorporated into the schedule at least 2 days per week. An anti-atherogenic diet should be followed, by reducing intake of saturated fats, trans fats, and cholesterol. Official recommendations are for saturated fat to comprise <7% of total calories and total fat 25–35% of total calories. Dietary fat should be mostly unsaturated and intake of simple sugar should be limited [1]. Medications may be initiated as adjunctive therapy to lifestyle changes in order to lower LDL-C levels and decrease blood pressure. Aspirin might be added prophylactically for patients at high risk for atherosclerotic cardiovascular disease (ASCVD) [1].

Outcome

This patient sees a dietician who starts him on a plan that is in accordance with AHA/NHBLI guidelines, trying to minimize saturated fats and cholesterol in his diet. He starts to cook at home instead of visiting fast-food restaurants. He starts to take short walks on his lunch break in order to incorporate some exercise into his day. After he starts to lose weight, his blood pressure is better controlled, and although he remains on medications, he avoids adding a third agent. On repeat labs, there is an improvement in HDL-C and LDL-C levels. He follows up with his primary care physician, cardiologist, and obesity medicine specialist every 6–12 months in order to have his waist circumference measured and BMI calculated, in addition to other aspects of the routine history and physical examination.

Clinical Pearls and Pitfalls

- An initial assessment of a patient with obesity or components of the metabolic syndrome must include the calculation of BMI and measurement of waist circumference.

- Initial assessment of obesity and metabolic syndrome must also include a complete medical history, family history, diet and lifestyle history, and a comprehensive set of blood tests including (but not limited to) a fasting lipid panel, glucose, and basic metabolic panel.
- Patients who fall in the overweight or obese range are at risk for cardiovascular disease (CVD), and those who have BMI >30 are at elevated mortality risk from all causes.
- Modest weight loss of 3–5% can be clinically significant and decrease a patient's risk of developing type 2 diabetes.
- Treatment of the metabolic syndrome includes addressing lifestyle, such as diet and exercise, and considering lipid-lowering therapy or antihypertensive therapy when indicated.

References

1. Grundy SM, Cleeman JI, Daniels SR, Donato KA, Eckel RH, Franklin BA, et al. Diagnosis and management of the metabolic syndrome: an American Heart Association/National Heart, Lung, and Blood Institute Scientific Statement. Circulation. 2005;112(17):2735–52. https://doi.org/10.1161/circulationaha.105.169404.
2. Jensen MD, Ryan DH, Apovian CM, Ard JD, Comuzzie AG, Donato KA, et al. 2013 AHA/ACC/TOS guideline for the management of overweight and obesity in adults. J Am Coll Cardiol. 2014;63:2985–3023. https://doi.org/10.1016/j.jacc.2013.11.004.
3. National Institute for Health and Clinical Excellence (NICE) guidelines. BMI: preventing ill health and premature death in black, Asian and other minority ethnic groups. July 2013. https://www.nice.org.uk/advice/lgb13.
4. National Institutes of Health/National Heart, Lung, and Blood Institute. Managing overweight and obesity in adults: systematic evidence review from the obesity expert

panel. Nov 2013. https://www.nhlbi.nih.gov/health-topics/managing-overweight-obesity-in-adults.

5. International Diabetes Foundation. The IDF consensus worldwide definition of the metabolic syndrome. 2016.
6. Lemieux I, Pascot A, Couillard C, Lamarche B, Tchernof A, Almeras N, Bergeron J, Gaudet D, Tremblay G, Prud'homme D, Nadeau A, Despres JP. Hypertriglyceridemic waist: a marker of the atherogenic metabolic triad (hyperinsulinemia; hyperapolipoprotein B; small, dense LDL) in men? Circulation. 2000;102:179.
7. Carr DB, Utzschneider KM, Hull RL, Kodama K, Retzlaff BM, Brunzell JD, Shofer JB, Fish BE, Knopp RH, Kahn SE. Intra-abdominal fat is a major determinant of the National Cholesterol Education Program Adult Treatment Panel III criteria for the metabolic syndrome. Diabetes. 2004;53:2087–94.
8. Park Y, Zhu S, Palaniappan L, et al. The metabolic syndrome: prevalence and associated risk factor findings in the US population from the Third National Health and Nutrition Examination Survey, 1988–1994. Arch Intern Med. 2003;163(4):427–36.
9. Palaniappan L, Carnethon M, Wang Y, et al. Predictors of the incident metabolic syndrome in adults: the insulin resistance atherosclerosis study. Diabetes Care. 2004;27(3):788–93.
10. Gennuso K, Gangnon R, Thraen-Borowski K, et al. Dose-response relationships between sedentary behaviour and the metabolic syndrome and its components. Diabetologia. 2015;58(3):485–92.
11. Green A, Jacques P, Rogers G, et al. Sugar-sweetened beverages and prevalence of the metabolically abnormal phenotype in the Framingham heart study. Obesity (Silver Spring). 2014;22(5):E157–63. https://doi.org/10.1002/oby.20724.
12. Pankow J, Jacobs D, Steinberger J, et al. Insulin resistance and cardiovascular disease risk factors in children of parents with the insulin resistance (metabolic) syndrome. Diabetes Care. 2004;27(3):775–80.
13. Mills G, Avery P, McCarthy M, et al. Heritability estimates for beta cell function and features of the insulin resistance syndrome in UK families with an increased susceptibility to type 2 diabetes. Diabetologia. 2004;47(4):732–8.
14. Van Tilburg J, Wijmenga C, van Haeften T, et al. A genome scan for loci linked to quantitative insulin traits in persons without diabetes: the Framingham offspring study. Diabetologia. 2003;46(11):1588.

Chapter 2
Identifying Comorbidities of Obesity

Caroline A. Andrew

Case Presentation

A 55-year-old woman presents to an obesity medicine specialist for evaluation. Her BMI is 37 kg/m^2. She has tried multiple diets in the past, with some success, but finds that she always regains the weight she loses. Her past medical history is significant for hypertension, for which she takes metoprolol and hydrochlorothiazide. She has osteoarthritis in her knees and is planning to have knee replacement surgery in a few months. For knee pain she takes ibuprofen daily. On further questioning, she reveals that she has not been sleeping well. Her husband complains that she snores. She wakes up multiple times throughout the night, does not feel well rested in the morning, and falls asleep at her desk occasionally in the afternoon. She has been taking diphenhydramine occasionally to help her fall asleep at night.

Review of symptoms is negative for chest pain, palpitations, shortness of breath, and lower extremity edema. Vitals: T 37.6, BP 140/80, HR 68, RR 12, and O2 98%. Exam is notable for crepitus in both knees, no evidence of effusions. Routine labs, including CMP, CBC, and HbA1c, are within normal limits.

C. A. Andrew (✉)
Hospital for Special Surgery, New York, NY, USA
e-mail: andrewca@hss.edu

L. J. Aronne, R. B. Kumar (eds.), *Obesity Management*,
https://doi.org/10.1007/978-3-030-01039-3_2

Assessment and Diagnosis

This patient has class 2 obesity (BMI 35–39.9 kg/m^2). She also suffers from HTN and osteoarthritis and, based on her history, may carry a diagnosis of obstructive sleep apnea (OSA), a common comorbidity of obesity. The prevalence of comorbidities in people with obesity has been found to be correlated with the degree of obesity. The odds of having multiple comorbidities increases significantly with each class of obesity [1].

OSA is a disorder defined by episodes of airway obstruction that affect ventilation during sleep [2]. Features of the condition include intermittent hypoxia and hypercapnia, interrupted sleep, daytime sleepiness, loud snoring, changes in intrathoracic pressure, and increased sympathetic nervous system activity [3]. Obesity is a risk factor for OSA. The adipose tissue creates a mechanical effect and pressure on the upper airway, causing pharyngeal narrowing and reducing lung volumes. Obesity can also affect the central nervous system (CNS) through adipokines and adipocyte-binding proteins that affect respiratory neuromuscular control [4]. The prevalence of OSA has been estimated to be 14% of men and 5% of women [5]. The prevalence is much higher among the population with overweight and obesity; it is estimated to be 70–80% among patients being evaluated for bariatric surgery [6].

The American Academy of Sleep Medicine recommends obtaining a detailed sleep history from any patient in whom obstructive sleep apnea is suspected. The physician should ask about snoring, witnessed apneic events, choking or gasping behavior at night, restlessness, and daytime sleepiness. There are several screening questionnaires that can also help a provider identify who might be at risk. The Epworth sleepiness scale is one that is commonly used, although there is a lack of evidence supporting its sensitivity and specificity [2]. Polysomnography is the gold standard diagnostic test for OSA and should be ordered for any patient in whom OSA is suspected. OSA is diagnosed with an obstructive respiratory disturbance index (RDI) >15 events per hour with or without symptoms or an obstructive RDI between 5 and 14 events per hour with symptoms [3, 7].

The treatment of OSA involves positive airway pressure therapy, most commonly provided by continuous positive airway pressure (CPAP). The CPAP maintains a positive pharyngeal transmural pressure, greater than the surrounding pressure, to preserve the airway space and prevent upper airway collapse. The use of positive airway pressure therapy has been shown to reduce the number of nocturnal respiratory events, decrease daytime sleepiness, improve blood pressure, and improve quality of life [8, 9].

Osteoarthritis is another common comorbidity associated with obesity. Although OA has a multifactorial etiology, it is well known that increased weight creates a mechanical stress on the joints, causing breakdown of cartilage, in particular in the knees and hips [10]. However, there has been found to be obesity-related arthritis in non-weight bearing joints, such as the hands, implying the involvement of systemic inflammation and circulating cytokines associated with adipose tissue affecting the joints [10, 11]. The American College of Rheumatology recommends weight loss for people who are overweight or obese in the treatment of knee and hip osteoarthritis [12].

Obesity also increases a patient's risk of developing HTN. The prevalence of HTN has been shown to increase with each class of obesity [13, 14]. This patient is already taking two antihypertensives, and her blood pressure is above the target range in the office.

This patient is also taking medications that may contribute to weight gain. Multiple prescription and over-the-counter medications have been associated with weight gain. For example, the patient's medication metoprolol, as a beta adrenergic receptor blocker, decreases energy expenditure and can be associated with weight gain [15]. Other medications may cause an increase in energy intake, such as antipsychotics and steroid hormones, or a decrease in energy expenditure, as can be seen in certain diabetes medications [2, 16]. Diphenhydramine, a member of the antihistamine class of medications, can also affect weight. Intravascular administration of histamine reduced food intake in animal studies, and histamine antagonism caused increased food intake [17, 18]. If possible, this class of drugs should be avoided in patients who have obesity and are trying to lose weight Table 2.1.

Table 2.1 Drug-Induced weight gain

Therapeutic category	Drug class	May cause weight gain	Alternatives that cause less weight gain, weight loss, or are weight neutral
Psychiatry	Antipsychotic	Clozapine Risperidone Olanzapine Quetiapine Other	Ziprasidone Aripiprazole
	Antidepressants and mood stabilizers	Citalopram Escitalopram Fluvoxamine Lithium MAOIs	Bupropion Nefazodone Fluoxetine (short term: <1 year) Sertraline (short term: <1 year)
Neurology	Anticonvulsants	Carbamazepine Gabapentin Valproate	Lamotrigine Topiramate Zonisamide
Endocrinology	Diabetes treatments	Insulin Sulfonylureas Thiazolidinedione	Metformin Acarbose Miglitol

Obstetrics and gynecology	Oral contraceptives	Progestational steroids Hormonal contraceptives containing progestational steroids	Barrier methods IUDs
	Endometriosis treatment	Depot leuprolide acetate	Surgical methods
Cardiology	Antihypertensives	α-blocker β-blocker	ACE inhibitors Calcium channel blockers
Infectious disease	Antiretroviral therapy	Protease inhibitors	None
General	Steroid hormones	Corticosteroids Progestational steroids	NSAIDs
	Antihistamines/ anticholinergics	Diphenhydramine Doxepin Cyproheptadine Other potent antihistamines	Decongestants Steroid inhalers

Management

First, this patient should be referred for polysomnography for further workup of possible OSA. Treatment of OSA will not only improve her symptoms of daytime sleepiness but could potentially treat her blood pressure. Weight loss can help address all of her comorbidities. Establishing a diet and exercise plan for weight loss may help improve her knee pain related to osteoarthritis. As metoprolol has been associated with weight gain, she should be switched to a weight-neutral medication for high blood pressure, such as an angiotensin-converting-enzyme (ACE) inhibitor, angiotensin receptor blocker (ARB), or calcium channel blocker (CCB). She should avoid taking diphenhydramine to help her fall asleep in order to prevent any further drug-induced weight gain [19].

Outcome

The patient is diagnosed with OSA and begins to use a CPAP nightly. She finds that she now feels much more rested when she wakes up in the morning and is no longer falling asleep at work. She stops using diphenhydramine and starts taking lisinopril instead of metoprolol. As she begins to lose weight, her knee pain improves and she is able to start walking for exercise.

References

1. Booth HP, Prevost AT, Gulliford MC. Impact of body mass index on prevalence of multimorbidity in primary care: cohort study. Fam Pract. 2014;31(1):38–43.
2. Sharma AM, Pischon T, Hardt S, et al. Hypothesis: beta-adrenergic receptor blockers and weight gain: a systematic analysis. Hypertension. 2001;37(2):250–4.
3. Kapur VK, Auckley DH, Chowdhuri S, et al. Clinical practice guideline for diagnostic testing for adult obstructive sleep

Clinical Pearls and Pitfalls

- The odds of having multiple comorbidities increases significantly with each class of obesity.
- OSA, a common comorbidity associated with obesity, is a disorder defined by episodes of airway obstruction that affect ventilation during sleep.
- Polysomnography is the gold standard diagnostic test for OSA and should be ordered for any patient in whom OSA is suspected.
- It is important to take a thorough history when assessing a patient with obesity, including a complete and detailed medication history, as certain classes of medications can be associated with weight gain.

apnea: an American academy of sleep medicine clinical practice guideline. J Clin Sleep Med. 2017;13(3):479–504. https://doi.org/10.5664/jcsm.6506.

4. Schwartz AR, Patil SP, Laffan AM, et al. Obesity and obstructive sleep apnea—pathogenic mechanisms and therapeutic approaches. Proc Am Thorac Soc. 2008;5:185–92.
5. Peppard PE, Young T, Barnet JH, Palta M, Hagen EW, Hla KM. Increased prevalence of sleep-disordered breathing in adults. Am J Epidemiol. 2013;177(9):1006–14.
6. Ravesloot MJ, van Maanen JP, Hilgevoord AA, van Wagensveld BA, de Vries N. Obstructive sleep apnea is underrecognized and underdiagnosed in patients undergoing bariatric surgery. Eur Arch Otorhinolaryngol. 2012;269(7):1865–71.
7. Berry RB, Budhiraja R, Gottlieb DJ, et al. Rules for scoring respiratory events in sleep: update of the 2007 AASM manual for the scoring of sleep and associated events. Deliberations of the sleep apnea definitions task force of the American academy of sleep medicine. J Clin Sleep Med. 2012;8(5):597–619. https://doi.org/10.5664/jcsm.2172.
8. Jonas D, Amick H, Feltner C, et al. Screening for obstructive sleep apnea in adults: evidence eeport and systematic review for the US preventive services task force. AHRQ Publication No. 14-05216-EF-1 2017.

9. Giles TL, Lasserson TJ, Smith BJ, et al. Continuous positive airways pressure for obstructive sleep apnoea in adults. Cochrane Database Syst Rev. 2006;1:CD001106.
10. Sellam J, Berenbaum F. Is osteoarthritis a metabolic disease? Joint Bone Spine. 2013;80(6):568–73.
11. Sowers MR, Karvonen-Gutierrez CA. The evolving role of obesity in knee osteoarthritis. Curr Opin Rheumatol. 2010;22:533–7.
12. Hochberg M, Altman R, April KT, et al. American College of rheumatology 2012 recommendations for the use of nonpharmacologic and pharmacologic therapies in osteoarthritis of the hand, hip, and knee. Arthritis Care Res. 2012;64(4):465–74.
13. Benjamin EJ, Blaha MJ, Chiuve SE, et al. Heart disease and stroke statistics-2017 update: a report from the American heart association. Circulation. 2017;135(10):e146–603.
14. Nguyen NT, Magno CP, Lane KT, et al. Association of hypertension, diabetes, dyslipidemia, and metabolic syndrome with obesity: findings from the National Health and Nutrition Examination Survey, 1999 to 2004. J Am Coll Surg. 2008;207(6):928–34.
15. Leslie WS, Hankey CR, Lean ME. Weight gain as an adverse effect of some commonly prescribed drugs: a systematic review. QJM. 2007;100(7):395–404.
16. Pijl H, Meinders AE. Bodyweight changes as an adverse effect of drug treatment. Drug Saf. 1996;14:329–42.
17. Kalucy RD. Drug-induced weight gain. Drugs. 1980;19(4):268–78.
18. Ratliff JC, Barber JA, Palmese LB, et al. Association of prescription H1 antihistamine use with obesity: results from the National Health and Nutrition Examination Survey. Obesity (Silver Spring). 2010;18(12):2398–400.
19. Saunders KH, Igel LI, Shukla AP, Aronne LJ. Drug induced weight gain: rethinking our choices. J Fam Pract. 2016;65(11):780–8.

Part II
Insulin Resistance Syndromes

Chapter 3
A Patient with High Cardiometabolic Risk

Alpana Shukla and Lindsay Mandel

Case Presentation

A 30-year-old South Asian male presents for an annual health exam. He denies any specific systemic complaints but admits to feeling somewhat run down lately, which he attributes to his work stress. Although never considered overweight, he has gained 5–6 lb over the past year, which came to his attention when his pants size increased. He has no significant past medical history. He has a positive family history for type 2 diabetes in his father and paternal grandfather, and premature coronary artery disease in his father, who had a CABG for triple vessel disease at the age of 50. He doesn't smoke and consumes four to five alcoholic drinks per week. He is lacto-ovo vegetarian, and his diet is heavy on carbohydrates. He has cereal for breakfast; a sandwich, pizza, or pasta for lunch; and a traditional, Indian meal at night which

A. Shukla (✉)
Comprehensive Weight Control Center, Division of Endocrinology, Diabetes and Metabolism, Weill Cornell Medical College, New York, NY, USA
e-mail: aps2004@med.cornell.edu

L. Mandel
Weill Cornell Medical College, New York, NY, USA

L. J. Aronne, R. B. Kumar (eds.), *Obesity Management*,
https://doi.org/10.1007/978-3-030-01039-3_3

includes half a plate of rice. He does not do structured exercise besides walking. On examination, his weight is 168 lb, BMI 24.8 kg/m^2, waist circumference 93 cm, and BP 126/80 mmHg. He has acanthosis nigricans around his neck. Systemic exam is within normal limits. Laboratory data show the following abnormalities: FBS 105, HbA1c 6.2%, triglycerides 200 mg/dl, HDL 36 mg/dl, and hsCRP 3 mg/dl.

Assessment and Diagnosis

This is a 30-year-old male patient with central adiposity, prediabetes, and dyslipidemia and a strong family history of premature cardiovascular disease.

In general, BMI ≥25 kg/m^2 is considered a risk factor for diabetes, and most, but not all, patients with T2DM are overweight or obese. However, data suggest that the BMI cut-point should be lower in ethnic groups with increased risk, and a BMI of ≥23 kg/m^2 should be used to define an increased risk in Asian Americans [1]. In fact, half of diabetes in Asian Americans is undiagnosed, which underscores the need to test at lower BMI thresholds in high-risk ethnic populations [2]. Although this patient is not overweight by traditional weight criteria, his waist circumference indicates an increased percentage of body fat distributed in the abdominal region. The clinically used ATP III guidelines suggest the presence of abdominal obesity if the waist circumference is ≥102 cm in men and ≥88 cm in women [3]. There is evidence, however, that certain ethnic groups are predisposed to metabolic complications at even lower waist circumferences. For this reason, the International Diabetes Federation guidelines suggest lower cut-points for abdominal obesity for certain ethnic groups, with cut-point ≥94 cm in men and ≥80 cm in women for Europids and ≥90 cm in males and ≥80 cm in females for South Asians, Chinese, Japanese, and Central Americans [4]. While the correlation between BMI and metabolic complications is certainly positive, for any given BMI measurement, an individual's risk for metabolic complications of obesity can vary based on differences in age, fitness, and distribution of body fat. Abdominal obesity, which tends to have a greater visceral component than that in the lower body which tends to be more subcutaneous, is associated with insulin resistance largely due to changes in the function of adipose tissue when viscerally accumulated [5]. Thus, increased abdominal girth on physical exam, even in the presence of a normal BMI, is a significant risk factor for the development of metabolic complications. The waist-to-hip ratio (WHR), defined as waist circumference divided by hip circumference, has also been used as an additional measurement of abdominal obesity (>0.90 for males and >0.85 for females) and may be a more efficient predictor of mortality in persons >75 years of age [6, 7]. Another clinical marker of insulin resistance, as evidenced in this patient, is acanthosis nigricans, a velvety, hyperpigmented thickening of the skin usually present in the axilla, groin, and neck regions.

This patient has low HDL and high triglyceride levels that are typical of dyslipidemia associated with insulin resistance and visceral adiposity. Although this patient has normal LDL levels on the standard lipid panel, a detailed lipoprotein profile may show a preponderance of atherogenic small dense LDL. The mildly elevated CRP is consistent with the proinflammatory milieu in obesity and in particular, visceral adiposity. Several studies have shown higher hsCRP levels in South Asians compared with other ethnic groups. These differences correlate with prevalence of metabolic syndrome and cardiovascular disease [8–10].

Lifestyle interventions are key to the management of prediabetes and associated metabolic comorbidities to prevent progression to diabetes and reduce risk of cardiovascular disease. Several studies in a variety of populations have confirmed the effectiveness of this strategy [11–14]. The Diabetes Prevention Program (DPP) was a landmark trial investigating whether intensive lifestyle modification or metformin could prevent or delay the onset of type 2 diabetes in individuals with impaired glucose tolerance. Participants in the intensive lifestyle intervention arm consisting of dietary modification with moderate physical exercise to achieve 7% weight loss lowered their risk of developing diabetes by 58%

compared with the control group that received placebo. The arm that received metformin with no lifestyle intervention saw a risk reduction of 31% compared to placebo [11]. The impact of these interventions in the South Asian population has been shown to be favorable, albeit of a lesser magnitude. The relative risk reduction over a median follow-up period of 30 months was 28.5% with lifestyle modification, 26.4% with metformin, and 28.2% with lifestyle modification plus metformin as compared with the control group in the Indian Diabetes Prevention Programme [12]. Long-term follow-up of three large studies of lifestyle intervention in patients with prediabetes has shown sustained reduction in the rate of conversion to type 2 diabetes: 43% reduction at 20 years in the Da Qing study [13], 43% reduction at 7 years in the Finnish Diabetes Prevention Study (DPS) [14], and 34% reduction at 10 years and 27% at 15 years in the US Diabetes Prevention Program Outcomes Study (DPPOS) [15, 16].

Apart from metformin, other pharmacologic agents that have been shown to decrease incident diabetes with variable efficacy include GLP-1 receptor agonists, orlistat, acarbose, and thiazolidinediones [17–22]. Currently, no pharmacologic therapy is FDA approved for prevention of diabetes. Given the strong evidence for long-term safety and efficacy, metformin is the recommended pharmacotherapeutic option in high-risk individuals with prediabetes, including those with BMI ≥35 kg/m^2, those aged <60 years, and women with prior gestational diabetes mellitus [22].

An aggressive approach is warranted in this patient at high risk of developing diabetes and cardiovascular disease and may include both lifestyle modification and metformin. The results of the DPP show that intensive lifestyle modification including frequent provider visits was efficacious in preventing the development of diabetes. However, for the patient in this vignette who has a very busy lifestyle, finding time to schedule frequent counseling sessions with a dietitian may not be practically feasible. Electronic and mobile health-based modalities to deliver core components of the DPP program may be considered in this patient, as several studies have demonstrated their effectiveness alongside more traditional face-to-face and coach-driven programs [23].

Management

The patient attended his first visit with a physician and dietitian in person. The patient was counseled to follow a low glycemic diet and engage in moderate-intensity physical activity for at least 150 min/week, since moderate-intensity physical activity has been shown to improve insulin sensitivity, reduce abdominal fat in young adults, and increase levels of HDL cholesterol [24]. He was encouraged to break up prolonged sedentary time, as this strategy can lower postprandial glucose levels [25]. Key components of nutrition counseling included advice on incorporating more protein and vegetables in the meals, reducing overall carbohydrate intake, and consuming carbohydrate portions at the end of the meal after protein and vegetables. This strategy of sequential macronutrient consumption, denoted "food order," has been demonstrated by our group and others to improve postprandial glucose regulation [26, 27] (Fig. 3.1). Given this patient's proclivity for carbohydrates, adherence to a low-carbohydrate diet may be a challenge. The glycemic effects of carbohydrate intake can be partly mitigated by the food order strategy. He participated in

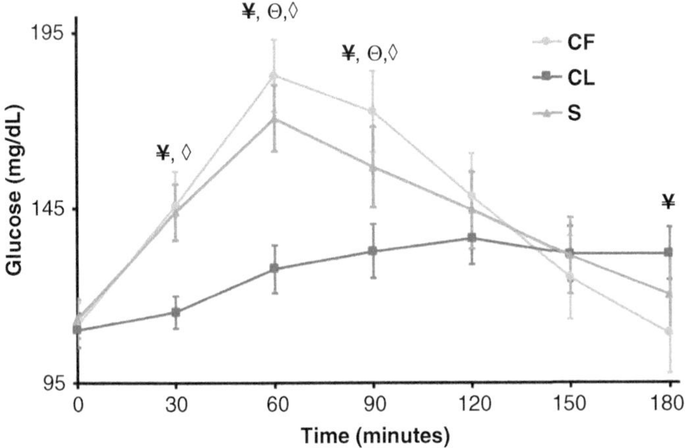

FIGURE 3.1 Postprandial glucose levels following carbohydrate-first (CF), carbohydrate-last (CL) and sandwich (S) meal orders (Shukla et al. [26])

monthly phone calls with a dietitian and was given access to BMIQ [28], an online weight management program incorporating the core components of the DPP and included remote electronic weight monitoring. In addition, the patient was prescribed metformin ER 500 mg once daily which was increased after a week to a dose of 1000 mg after breakfast.

Outcome

He returned for an in-person follow-up at 6 months. He reported developing some bloating and diarrhea at first on metformin, but the side effects abated after a week or two. He made several changes in his diet and was able to incorporate the food order strategy during 50% or more of his meals. His weight was down by 13 lb, and he reported feeling more energetic. His weight was 155 lb, BMI 22.9, waist circumference 88 cm, and BP 120/76. HbA1c was 5.6%. At 1-year follow-up, his weight had further reduced to 150 lb and waist circumference to 85 cm. HbA1c was 5.5%, triglycerides 140 mg/dl, HDL 42 mg/dl, and hsCRP 0.8 mg/dl.

Clinical Pearls and Pitfalls

- High-risk ethnic populations such as South Asians are predisposed to develop metabolic syndrome and type 2 diabetes at lower BMIs due to variation in body fat distribution, so measures of central adiposity like waist circumference may be better for risk assessment.
- Intensive lifestyle modification has been shown to significantly decrease the risk of progression to diabetes and can be combined with metformin therapy in high-risk individuals.
- Lifestyle modification needs to be individualized, and remote internet-based lifestyle interventions in conjunction with telephonic Dietitian support are a feasible and effective strategy for individuals unable to attend frequent clinic visits.

References

1. WHO Expert Consultation. Appropriate body-mass index for Asian populations and its implications for policy and intervention strategies. Lancet. 2004;363:157–63.
2. Menke A, Casagrande S, Geiss L, Cowie CC. Prevalence of and trends in diabetes among adults in the United States, 1988–2012. JAMA. 2015;314:1021–9.
3. National Cholesterol Education Program (NCEP) Expert Panel on Detection, Evaluation, and Treatment of High Blood Cholesterol in Adults (Adult Treatment Panel III). Third report of the National Cholesterol Education Program (NCEP) expert panel on detection, evaluation, and treatment of high blood cholesterol in adults (adult treatment panel III) final report. Circulation. 2002;106(25):3143–421.
4. International Diabetes Federation. The IDF consensus worldwide definition of metabolic syndrome. Brussels. 2006.
5. Westphal SA. Obesity, abdominal obesity, and insulin resistance. Clin Cornerstone. 2008;9(1):23–9. discussion 30–31
6. Price GM, Uauy R, Breeze E, Bulpitt CJ, Fletcher AE. Weight, shape, and mortality risk in older persons: elevated waist-hip ratio, not high body mass index, is associated with a greater risk of death. Am J Clin Nutr. 2006;84(2):449–60.
7. World Health Organization. Report of a WHO expert consultation. Waist circumference and waist-hip ratio. Geneva, Switzerland: 2008.
8. Chambers JC, Eda S, Bassett P, Karim Y, Thompson SG, Gallimore R, Pepys MB, Kooner JS. C-reactive protein, insulin resistance, central obesity, and coronary heart disease risk in Indian Asians from the United Kingdom compared with European whites. Circulation. 2001;104:145–15.
9. Forouhi NG, Sattar N, McKeigue PM. Relation of C-reactive protein in body fat distribution and features of the metabolic syndrome in Europeans and South Asians. Int J Obes Relat Metab Disord. 2001;25:1327–31.
10. Anand SS, Razak F, Yi Q, Davis B, Jacobs R, Vuksan V, Lonn E, Teo K, McQueen M, Yusuf S. C-reactive protein as a screening test for cardiovascular risk in a multiethnic population. Arterioscler Thromb Vasc Biol. 2004;24:1509–15.
11. Knowler WC, Barrett-Connor E, Fowler SE, Hamman RF, Lachin JM, Walker EA, Nathan DM, and Diabetes Prevention Program Research Group. Reduction in the incidence of type 2 diabetes with lifestyle intervention or metformin. N Engl J Med. 2002;346(6):393–403.

12. Ramachandran A, Snehalatha C, Mary S, Mukesh B, Bhaskar AD, Vijay V. Indian Diabetes Prevention Programme (IDPP). The Indian Diabetes Prevention Programme shows that lifestyle modification and metformin prevent type 2 diabetes in Asian Indian subjects with impaired glucose tolerance (IDPP-1). Diabetologia. 2006;49(2):289–97.
13. Li G, Zhang P, Wang J, et al. The long-term effect of lifestyle interventions to prevent diabetes in the China Da Qing diabetes prevention study: a 20-year follow-up study. Lancet. 2008;371:1783–9.
14. Lindström J, Ilanne-Parikka P, Peltonen M, et al. Finnish diabetes prevention study group. Sustained reduction in the incidence of type 2 diabetes by lifestyle intervention: follow-up of the Finnish diabetes prevention study. Lancet. 2006;368:1673–9.
15. Knowler WC, Fowler SE, Hamman RF, et al. Diabetes prevention program research group. 10-year follow-up of diabetes incidence and weight loss in the diabetes prevention program outcomes study. Lancet. 2009;374:1677–86.
16. Nathan DM, Barrett-Connor E, Crandall JP, et al. Long-term effects of lifestyle intervention or metformin on diabetes development and microvascular complications: the DPP outcomes study. Lancet Diabetes Endocrinol. 2015;3:866–75.
17. Chiasson J-L, Josse RG, Gomis R, Hanefeld M, Karasik A, Laakso M, STOP-NIDDM Trial Research Group. Acarbose for prevention of type 2 diabetes mellitus: the STOP-NIDDM randomised trial. Lancet. 2002;359:2072–7.
18. Torgerson JS, Hauptman J, Boldrin MN, Sjöström L. XENical in the prevention of diabetes in obese subjects (XENDOS) study: a randomized study of orlistat as an adjunct to lifestyle changes for the prevention of type 2 diabetes in obese patients. Diabetes Care. 2004;27:155–61.
19. le Roux CW, Astrup A, Fujioka K, et al. SCALE obesity prediabetes NN8022-1839 study group. 3 years of liraglutide versus placebo for type 2 diabetes risk reduction and weight management in individuals with prediabetes: a randomised, double-blind trial. Lancet. 2017;389:1399–409.
20. Gerstein HC, Yusuf S, Bosch J, et al. DREAM (Diabetes REduction Assessment with ramipril and rosiglitazone Medication) trial investigators. Effect of rosiglitazone on the frequency of diabetes in patients with impaired glucose tolerance or impaired fasting glucose: a randomised controlled trial. Lancet. 2006;368:1096–105.

21. DeFronzo RA, Tripathy D, Schwenke DC, et al. ACT NOW study. pioglitazone for diabetes prevention in impaired glucose tolerance. N Engl J Med. 2011;364:1104–15.
22. Diabetes Prevention Program Research Group. Long-term safety, tolerability, and weight loss associated with metformin in the diabetes prevention program outcomes study. Diabetes Care. 2012;35:731–7.
23. American Diabetes Association Standards of Medical Care in Diabetes-2018. Prevention or delay of type 2 diabetes. Diabetes Care. 2018;41(Supplement 1):S51–4.
24. Fedewa MV, Gist NH, Evans EM, Dishman RK. Exercise and insulin resistance in youth: a meta-analysis. Pediatrics. 2014;133:e163–74.
25. Thorp AA, Kingwell BA, Sethi P, Hammond L, Owen N, Dunstan DW. Alternating bouts of sitting and standing attenuate postprandial glucose responses. Med Sci Sports Exerc. 2014;46:2053–61.
26. Shukla AP, Andono J, Touhamy SH, et al. Carbohydrate-last meal pattern lowers postprandial glucose and insulin excursions in type 2 diabetes. BMJ Open Diabetes Research and Care. 2017;5:e000440. https://doi.org/10.1136/bmjdrc-2017-000440.
27. Imai S, Fukui M, Kajiyama S. Effect of eating vegetables before carbohydrates on glucose excursions in patients with type 2 diabetes. J Clin Biochem Nutr. 2014;54(1):7–11.
28. www.bmiq.com.

Chapter 4
Polycystic Ovarian Syndrome

Alpana Shukla and Lindsay Mandel

Case Presentation

A 28-year-old female presents to her primary care doctor for concern of increased weight gain and amenorrhea. She has had irregular menses since menarche at 11 years of age. She has been intermittently on oral contraceptive pills (OCPs) in the past which regularized her menses, but she hasn't taken an OCP in the past 2 years. She was overweight as a teenager but has had a recent abrupt weight gain of 30 lbs in the past year. She has tried to lose weight with a low-fat diet and exercise in the past and lost 10 lbs 2 years ago, which she subsequently regained. Although her menses were irregular in the past, she would have 3–4 cycles/year, but now her last menstrual period was 6 months ago. Home pregnancy test is negative. She has always had facial hair which she has managed cosmetically by waxing, but she feels this has now

A. Shukla (✉)
Comprehensive Weight Control Center, Division of Endocrinology, Diabetes and Metabolism, Weill Cornell Medical College, New York, NY, USA
e-mail: aps2004@med.cornell.edu

L. Mandel
Weill Cornell Medical College, New York, NY, USA

L. J. Aronne, R. B. Kumar (eds.), *Obesity Management*,
https://doi.org/10.1007/978-3-030-01039-3_4

become excessive and darker over the past year. She has a family history of type 2 diabetes in her mother. She is not trying to conceive but she is anxious about her fertility in the future. Her physical examination is significant for a body mass index (BMI) of 32 kg/m^2, waist circumference 95 cm, BP 130/80, moderate hirsutism and acne, and acanthosis nigricans around the neck. She has no clinical stigmata suggestive of Cushing's syndrome. Laboratory tests reveal a total testosterone level of 60 ng/dl (reference range, 14–53 ng/dl), calculated free testosterone level of 15.3 pg/ml per milliliter (reference range, 0.6–6.8 pg per milliliter), TSH 3.5 μIU/ml, FBG 102 mg/dl, and HbA1c 5.7%.

Assessment and Diagnosis

The patient in the vignette has Class 1 obesity with central adiposity, prediabetes, and clinical and biochemical hyperandrogenism with oligomenorrhea suggestive of the polycystic ovary syndrome (PCOS).

While there are several definitions of PCOS, the most widely used Rotterdam criteria require at least two of the following otherwise unexplained abnormalities to make a diagnosis of PCOS: hyperandrogenism (clinical, biochemical, or both), ovulatory dysfunction, and polycystic ovarian morphologic features on ultrasound [1]. Clinical features of hyperandrogenism include acne, hirsutism (defined as excessive terminal hair that appears in a male pattern), and androgenic alopecia. Biochemical hyperandrogenism refers to an elevated serum androgen level and includes an elevated total, bioavailable, or free serum testosterone level with the most sensitive test for hyperandrogenemia in women with PCOS being free testosterone. Given the uncertain reliability of direct free testosterone assays, it is recommended to calculate free testosterone using measurements of total testosterone and sex hormone-binding globulin (SHBG) [2]. Ovulatory dysfunction may manifest as frequent bleeding at intervals less than 21 days or infrequent bleeding at intervals greater than 35 days. However, it is pertinent to note that 15–40% of women with hyperandrogenism and regular menses occurring at 21–35-day intervals have ovulatory dysfunction [3]. On ultrasound, polycystic ovaries are characterized by 12 or more antral follicles (2–9 mm in diameter) in either ovary, an ovarian volume that is greater than 10 (mL) in either ovary, or both [1]. It should be noted, however, that ultrasound findings lack specificity, as up to 70% of healthy young women may have polycystic ovaries on ultrasound [4].

This patient fulfills two of the three criteria, and therefore ovarian ultrasonography is not needed for diagnosis; however, disorders that can mimic PCOS such as hyperprolactinemia, hypothyroidism, and nonclassical congenital adrenal hyperplasia (CAH) should be excluded. 21-hydroxylase deficiency is the most common cause of nonclassical CAH which can be ruled out by an early morning follicular phase 17-OH progesterone level <2 ng/ml. Where clinically indicated (facial plethora, purple striae, proximal myopathy, easy bruising), Cushing's syndrome should be ruled out by measuring 24-h urinary free cortisol and late-night salivary cortisol or by an overnight dexamethasone suppression test.

The pathophysiology of PCOS is incompletely understood; however, data suggest a central role for insulin resistance in promoting hyperandrogenism and related metabolic comorbidities. Hyperinsulinemia increases bioavailable or free testosterone by inhibiting hepatic synthesis of SHBG and also promotes ovarian and adrenal androgen production [5]. It is currently estimated that between 50 and 70% of women with PCOS are obese [6, 7] with 30–35% having impaired glucose tolerance and 3–10% with type 2 diabetes mellitus [8]. The oral glucose tolerance test (OGTT) is recommended as the gold standard test to screen for IGT/T2DM. Measurement of fasting blood glucose level alone is not recommended, but HbA1c level may be acceptable if OGTT is not feasible [4, 8]. PCOS is associated with other conditions linked with insulin resistance and the metabolic syndrome such as central adiposity, dyslipidemia, hypertension, obstructive sleep apnea (OSA), and nonalcoholic steatohepatitis (NASH) [8–10]. A fasting lipid panel and measurement of waist circumference in addition to BMI and blood pressure is recommended in all patients [4]. In patients with symptoms suggestive of sleep apnea, further assessment with a polysomnogram is indicated. Routine screening for NASH is not currently recommended; however, women with PCOS and metabolic risk factors (as described in this vignette) may be screened using serum markers of liver dysfunction. If serum markers are elevated, further evaluation by ultrasound and liver biopsy may be considered. Routine measurements of serum insulin levels to assess insulin resistance are not recommended due to their uncertain clinical utility beyond what can be gleaned from clinical assessment of metabolic phenotype.

The hormonal disturbances that characterize PCOS can cause anovulatory menstrual cycles, leading to irregular menstrual periods, as seen in this patient. In fact, PCOS is often diagnosed in patients presenting for difficulties becoming pregnant and represents the most common cause of female infertility. Unopposed estrogen from anovulatory cycles without the action of progesterone from the corpus luteum is a risk factor for the development of endometrial hyperplasia. The risk of endometrial cancer is estimated to be 2.7 higher in women with PCOS as compared to women without PCOS [11].

Due to the complex nature of the disorder, the concerns of a patient with PCOS are multifactorial: she might present with any combination of menstrual irregularity, hirsutism, infertility, and metabolic complications such as obesity and insulin resistance. All of these conditions need to be considered in choosing treatment options, and whether the woman desires to become pregnant is of particular importance. For women who do not desire pregnancy in the near future, combined oral contraceptives (OCPs) are first line and work by suppressing gonadotropin secretion in the pituitary and subsequent ovarian androgen production as well as increasing SHBG to reduce free testosterone. While they do not address the underlying hormonal derangements in PCOS, OCPs can restore regularity to menstrual periods, reduce hirsutism, and reduce the risk of endometrial hyperplasia in addition to their contraceptive actions. Spironolactone, an androgen receptor antagonist, may be used as an add-on therapy to OCPs when hirsutism is inadequately treated. Topical eflornithine and mechanical methods are other options to manage hirsutism which can be used in combination with the above modalities.

Weight loss of 5–10% has been shown to reduce cardiometabolic risk factors, reduce androgen levels, and increase fertility. Lifestyle interventions including diet modification and increased physical activity are recommended as first-line therapy for all patients with overweight/obesity [4, 8, 11]. As a large proportion of patients with PCOS have insulin resistance, metformin is commonly used as it improves insulin resistance and may improve ovulatory function in patients with PCOS. It is recommended as second-line therapy for menstrual irregularity in women who cannot take or are intolerant to OCPs [8]. While the weight loss reported in systematic reviews and meta-analysis of metformin is modest (2.9%) [12], significant weight loss in combination with a low-glycemic diet has been observed in our clinical experience [13]. GLP-1 receptor analogs have been studied for weight reduction and glycemic control in patients with PCOS and have also been shown in some studies to improve androgen excess and increase menstruation frequency [14]. They may be considered as adjuncts for weight management in women who are not imminently considering pregnancy. Similarly, women with severe obesity are candidates for bariatric surgery, which is shown to improve fertility and other features associated with PCOS [15, 16].

While this patient is currently not planning pregnancy, this disease primarily affects women of child-bearing age, and thus treatment that restores fertility is often a consideration at some point during a patient's treatment. Clomiphene is considered to be the first-line agent for ovulation induction in women with PCOS, but it should be noted that pregnancy without medical assistance is common even among patients with complaints of infertility [17]. For women with PCOS who become pregnant, pregnancy is more likely to be complicated by gestational hypertension, diabetes, preeclampsia, and pregnancy loss, and these women may need increased surveillance during pregnancy [18]. The hyperinsulinemic state of PCOS can lead to macrosomia in the infant, and gestational weight gain should be limited to 15–25 lbs in women who are overweight and 11–20 lbs in women with obesity [19].

The management of this patient must address her current needs for menstrual regularity and treatment of hirsutism and acne, and optimize therapy to ameliorate the metabolic derangements and improve future fertility. She has tried a low-fat diet in the past with limited short-term results, which is not surprising given that complex weight regulating mechanisms oppose maintenance of a lower body weight. The addition of metformin to lifestyle modification is a reasonable approach in addition to an OCP. An incremental approach to optimize weight loss will improve metabolic comorbidities and also improve future fertility and may include additional weight loss pharmacotherapies.

Management

The patient received counseling from a registered dietitian at the initial visit and subsequently at 3 and 6 months. She adopted a low-glycemic diet and joined a gym, where she engaged in aerobic exercise combined with resistance training for 30–45 min, 5 days a week. Since she was not desiring pregnancy for the near future, she was started on Yasmin, a combined oral contraceptive containing drospirenone, a spironolactone analog as the progestin. She was also prescribed metformin 500 mg ER once daily which was increased at weekly intervals to a total dose of 1500 mg (1000 mg with breakfast and 500 mg with dinner).

Outcome

The patient returned for follow-up 6 months later. Her weight was down 6% from her initial visit with a current BMI of 30. Her acne had cleared and she reported slightly reduced facial hair. Monthly menses had resumed with the addition of OCPs, and at this point, the patient still did not desire pregnancy. She felt that her weight had plateaued with metformin and dietary modification for the past month. Liraglutide, a GLP-1 analog, was added to her regimen starting at 0.6 mg daily and increased to 1.2 mg after a week. The dose was further increased to 1.8 mg 6 weeks later. At her 1-year follow-up visit, her weight was down by 14%, BMI was 26 kg/m^2, and hirsutism was much improved. HbA1c was 5.6%. She now desired pregnancy, so Yasmin and liraglutide were discontinued, leaving her on metformin. She conceived 2 months later, and metformin was continued following a shared decision with the patient given her previous history of prediabetes and strong family history of T2DM.

Clinical Pearls and Pitfalls

- The diagnosis of PCOS requires two of the following three criteria to be fulfilled: clinical and/or biochemical hyperandrogenism, ovulatory dysfunction, and polycystic ovarian morphologic features on ultrasound as well as the exclusion of disorders that can mimic this syndrome (hypothyroidism, hyperprolactinemia, and nonclassical congenital adrenal hyperplasia).
- Insulin resistance is central to the etiology of PCOS, and consequently, women with PCOS have associated metabolic derangements and increased cardiovascular risk factors.
- The management of PCOS should be targeted to address patient-specific concerns, including menstrual irregularity, acne and hirsutism, and infertility concomitant with management of metabolic comorbidities.
- Lifestyle modification plays a key role in treatment, and weight loss of 5–10% in patients with overweight/obesity has been shown to reduce cardio-

metabolic risk factors, reduce androgen levels, and increase fertility.
- OCPs are first-line therapy for management of PCOS in women not planning pregnancy; they ameliorate hyperandrogenism, regularize menstrual cycles, and provide reliable endometrial protection and contraception.
- Metformin is a useful adjunct to lifestyle modification in women with impaired glucose tolerance who have failed lifestyle modification alone and may also induce weight loss and improve ovulatory function. It is a recommended second-line therapy for menstrual irregularity in women who cannot take or tolerate OCPs.
- Pharmacotherapies for obesity and bariatric surgery should be considered adjuncts for weight management in eligible patients.

References

1. The Rotterdam ESHRE/ASRM-Sponsored PCOS Consensus Workshop Group. Revised 2003 consensus on diagnostic criteria and long-term health risks related to polycystic ovary syndrome (PCOS). Hum Reprod. 2004;19:41–7.
2. Rosner W, Auchus RJ, Azziz R, Sluss PM, Raff H. Position statement: utility, limitations, and pitfalls in measuring testosterone: an endocrine society position statement. J Clin Endocrinol Metab. 2007;92:405–13.
3. Azziz R, Carmina E, Dewailly D, Diamanti-Kandarakis E, Escobar-Morreale HF, Futterweit W, Janssen OE, Legro RS, Norman RJ, Taylor AE, Witchel SF. The androgen excess and PCOS society criteria for the polycystic ovary syndrome: the complete task force report. Fertil Steril. 2009;91(2):456–88.
3. Kristensen S, Ramlau-Hansen CH, Ernst E, et al. A very large proportion of young Danish women have polycystic ovaries: is a revision of the Rotterdam criteria needed? Hum Reprod. 2010;25:3117–22.

4. ACOG Committee on Practice Bulletins--Gynecology. ACOG practice bulletin no. 108: polycystic ovary syndrome. Obstet Gynecol. 2009;114(4):936–49.
5. Azziz R, Woods KS, Reyna R, Key TJ, Knochenhauer ES, Yildiz BO. The prevalence and features of the polycystic ovary syndrome in an unselected population. J Clin Endocrinol Metab. 2004;89:2745–9.
6. Ehrmann DA. Polycystic ovary syndrome. N Engl J Med. 2005;352:1223–36.
7. Legro RS, Arslanian SA, Ehrmann DA, et al. Diagnosis and treatment of polycystic ovary syndrome: an Endocrine Society clinical practice guideline. J Clin Endocrinol Metab. 2013;98:4565–92.
8. Vgontzas AN, Legro RS, Bixler EO, Grayev A, Kales A, Chrousos GP. Polycystic ovary syndrome is associated with obstructive sleep apnea and daytime sleepiness: role of insulin resistance. J Clin Endocrinol Metab. 2001;86(2):517–20.
9. Hossain N, Stepanova M, Afendy A, Nader F, Younossi Y, Rafiq N, Goodman Z, Younossi ZM. Non-alcoholic steatohepatitis (NASH) in patients with polycystic ovarian syndrome (PCOS). Scand J Gastroenterol. 2011;46(4):479–84.
10. Dumesic DA, Lobo RA. Cancer risk and PCOS. Steroids. 2013;78:782–5.
11. Moran LJ, Pasquali R, Teede HJ, Hoeger KM, Norman RJ. Treatment of obesity in polycystic ovary syndrome: a position statement of the androgen excess and polycystic ovary syndrome society. Fertil Steril. 2009;92:1966–82.
12. Padwal R, Li SK, Lau DC. Long-term pharmacotherapy for over-weight and obesity: a systematic review and meta-analysis of randomized controlled trials. Int J Obes Relat Metab Disord. 2003;27:1437–46.
13. Mandel, L, Shukla A, Litman E, and Aronne L. The utility of metformin as antiobesity pharmacotherapy. Poster presented at: Obesity Week 2017; 2017 Oct 29–Nov 2; Washington DC.
14. Lamos EM, Malek R, Davis SN. GLP-1 receptor agonists in the treatment of polycystic ovary syndrome. Expert Rev Clin Pharmacol. 2017;10(4):401–8.
15. Butterworth J, Deguara J, Borg CM. Bariatric surgery, polycystic ovary syndrome, and infertility. J Obes. 2016;2016:1871594.
16. Skubleny D, Switzer NJ, Gill RS, Dykstra M, Shi X, Sagle MA, de Gara C, Birch DW, Karmali S. The impact of bariatric surgery on polycystic ovary syndrome: a systematic review and meta-analysis. Obes Surg. 2016;26(1):169–76.

17. McCartney CR, Marshall JC. Polycystic ovary syndrome. N Engl J Med. 2016;375(1):54–64.
18. Kamalanathan S, Sahoo JP, Sathyapalan T. Pregnancy in polycystic ovary syndrome. Indian J Endocrinol Metab. 2013;17(1):37–43.
19. American College of Obstetricians and Gynecologists. ACOG Committee opinion no. 548: weight gain during pregnancy. Obstet Gynecol. 2013;121:210–2.

Part III
Type II Diabetes and Obesity

Chapter 5
Diagnosing Type II Diabetes and Choosing Medications in Patients with Obesity

Rekha B. Kumar

Case Presentation

A 48-year-old female presents to her primary care doctor for an annual visit. She was told she had the metabolic syndrome at her physical 1 year ago when she had a hemoglobin A1c of 6.1%, hypertension (BP of 145/90), and hypertriglyceridemia (170 mg/dl). At that time, she was told of her risk of developing type II diabetes and advised to lose weight. Over the past year, the patient has gained 12 lbs and attributes her weight gain to stress and inability to prioritize a healthy diet due to balancing her career with taking care of her children. Her diet consists of high-fat and high-carbohydrate foods with fast food in the diet several times per week including processed baked goods and sugar-sweetened beverages with lunch and dinner. She has a desk job and drives back and forth to her

R. B. Kumar (✉)
Comprehensive Weight Control Center, Division of Endocrinology, Diabetes and Metabolism, Weill Cornell Medical College, New York, NY, USA
e-mail: reb9037@med.cornell.edu

L. J. Aronne, R. B. Kumar (eds.), *Obesity Management*,
https://doi.org/10.1007/978-3-030-01039-3_5

office with no additional structured exercise. She has a family history of obesity and type II diabetes in her maternal grandmother but reports that her parents are normal weight. She does not drink alcohol or smoke. She has two children and had diet-controlled gestational diabetes during her second pregnancy.

The patient's current medications include lisinopril 20 mg for hypertension, atorvastatin 20 mg for hyperlipidemia, and an omeprazole 40 mg for acid reflux.

Upon evaluation, she is found to have a fasting blood glucose of 141 mg/dl and a hemoglobin A1c of 6.7%. The patient is informed that she has developed type II diabetes and must start medication and lifestyle intervention. The patient's BMI is 33 kg/m^2, BP of 138/92, and P of 90. Her waist circumference is 39 inches. The rest of her laboratory evaluation is significant for an LDL of 130, HDL of 41, and AST of 52 units/L (10–40 U/L) and ALT of 65 units/L (7–56 U/L).

The physician informs the patient that her continued weight gain likely has contributed to the progression of her metabolic syndrome and prediabetes to type II diabetes. The physician expresses concern that she may have developed fatty liver as well based on her laboratory evaluation. The patient is agreeable to structured counseling on diet and exercise and inquiries about medicines that she could take to treat her diabetes.

Assessment and Diagnosis

This patient has a history of metabolic syndrome which is a risk factor for type II diabetes and cardiovascular disease such as heart attack and stroke. The components of the metabolic syndrome are impaired glucose tolerance (fasting blood glucose >100 mg/dl), low HDL cholesterol (< 50 mg/dl for women, < 40 mg/dl for men), elevated fasting triglycerides > 150 mg/dl, elevated blood pressure >130/85 mmHg, and increased waist circumference (>40 inches for men and > 35 inches for women) [1]. Meeting three of these criteria qualifies as having the metabolic syndrome. It is important to identify these risk factors in patients in order to properly counsel patients on managing their obesity. An algorithmic approach to diagnosing overweight and obesity has been outlined by 2013 guidelines proposed by the American Heart Association (AHA)/American College of Cardiology (ACC)/The Obesity Society (TOS) by Jensen et al. [2]. The AHA/ACC/TOS guidelines suggest assessing body mass index (BMI) to screen for overweight and obesity at each patient encounter. Assessment should include height, weight, and calculation of BMI. If a patient is found to have a normal BMI ($\geq$18.5–<25 kg/m^2), he or she should be advised to avoid weight gain, and potential risk factors for weight gain in their history should be addressed. If a patient meets criteria for overweight or obesity, the patient should be screened and treated for cardiovascular comorbidities, including diabetes, hypertension, and hyperlipidemia. The severity of obesity determined by BMI class and comorbidities should further lead the physician through the algorithm toward offering behavioral intervention for weight management or behavioral intervention with anti-obesity pharmacotherapy: if BMI exceeds 30 kg/m^2 or if BMI is greater than 27 kg/m^2 with comorbidities. Individuals with refractory class II obesity (BMI 35 to <40 kg/m^2) with medical complications, as well as with class III obesity (BMI $\geq$ 40 kg/m^2), should be offered bariatric surgical options.

This patient was informed of her metabolic syndrome, obesity, and risk of progressive disease at her prior visit. In the setting continued weight gain, she progressed to develop type II diabetes. The American Diabetes Association (ADA) criteria for the diagnosis of type II diabetes include any of the following [3]:

1. A fasting plasma glucose (FPG) level of 126 mg/dL (7 mmol/L) or higher (after at least 8 h of fasting.
2. A hemoglobin A1c (HbA1c) level of 6.5% or higher;the test should be performed in a laboratory using a method that is certified by the National Glycohemoglobin Standardization Program (NGSP) and standardized to the diabetes control and complications trial (DCCT) reference assay (ref).

3. A 2-h plasma glucose level of 200 mg/dL (11.1 mmol/L) or higher during a 75-g oral glucose tolerance test (OGTT).
4. A random plasma glucose of 200 mg/dL (11.1 mmol/L) or higher in a patient with symptoms of hyperglycemia (polyuria, polydipsia, blurry vision).

Management

The treatment of metabolic syndrome and prediabetes/impaired glucose tolerance should always focus on lifestyle intervention with a calorie-restricted, low-glycemic index diet and increased physical activity. In the Diabetes Prevention Program (DPP) study, beneficial changes in diet and physical activity significantly reduced the chances that a subject with prediabetes/impaired glucose tolerance would develop diabetes (58% reduction). Metformin also reduced risk, although to a lesser degree (31%) [4]. Once pharmacotherapy is necessary for type II diabetes, metformin is considered first-line therapy. Historically sulfonylureas and thiazolidinediones were considered second-line therapy, but with the increasing prevalence of obesity, several diabetes guidelines such as the American Association of Clinical Endocrinologists (AACE), the American College of Endocrinology (ACE), and the European Association for the Study of Diabetes (EASD) now recommend second-line agents that are weight neutral or stimulate weight loss (GLP1 RA's, SGLT2i's, DPP-4i's) as opposed to sulfonylureas and thiazolidinediones that may cause hunger and weight gain due to risk of hypoglycemia and compensatory self-treatment with increasing food intake and particularly carbohydrate intake [5] (Fig. 5.1).

Outcome

After the visit with her primary care doctor, the patient had a consultation with a registered dietitian who placed the patient on a low-glycemic diet (<100 grams of total carbohydrates/day), started tracking her food intake through a jour-

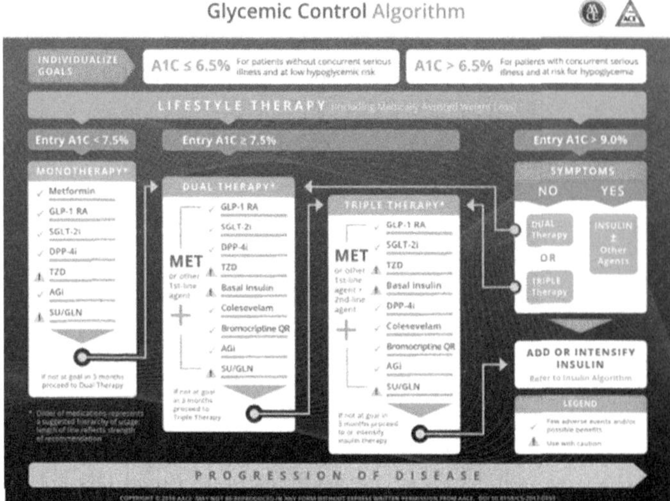

FIGURE 5.1 AACE/ACE diabetes algorithm 2018

nal, and started on metformin which was titrated to full dose of 1 g twice daily, but she did not tolerate the full dose due to gastrointestinal side effects. She was able to tolerate 1 g once daily so second-line therapy with the SGLT-2 inhibitor empagliflozin was initiated as per the AACE/ACE algorithm. Over the subsequent 4 months, patient lost 5% of her total body weight, hbA1c improved from 6.7 to 5.9%, and she felt motivated to slowly increase her physical activity as she saw results of the diet and medical therapy.

Clinical Pearls and Pitfalls

- Recognize features and screen for the metabolic syndrome, overweight, and obesity as risk factors for the development of type II diabetes.
- Be familiar with various diagnostic criteria for type II diabetes.

- Appreciate the efficacy of lifestyle and dietary intervention in prediabetes and impaired glucose tolerance (diabetes prevention program study).
- Metformin is a first-line therapy for diabetes, and even low doses can be beneficial if the full dose cannot be tolerated.
- Current guidelines for second-line agents after metformin for diabetes now emphasize medicines that are weight neutral or can stimulate weight loss such as GLP1 RA's, SGLT2i's, and DPP-4i's.
- Appreciate that there is improvement in metabolic health when patients lose 5–10% of their total body weight even when their BMI still qualifies as having overweight or obesity.

References

1. Motillo S, et al. The metabolic syndrome and cardiovascular risk a systematic review and meta-analysis. J Am Coll Cardiol. 2010;56(14):1113–32.
2. Jensen MD, et al. 2013 AHA/ACC/TOS guideline for the management of overweight and obesity in adults: a report of the American College of Cardiology/American Heart Association Task Force on Practice Guidelines and the Obesity Society. J Am Coll Cardiol. 2014;63(25 Pt B):2985–3023.
3. American Diabetes Association. Classification and diagnosis of diabetes: standards of medical care in diabetes-2018. Diabetes Care. 2018;41(Suppl 1):S13–27.
4. Diabetes Prevention Program Research Group. N Engl J Med. 2002;346:393–403. https://www.nejm.org/doi/full/10.1056/NEJMoa012512
5. Garber, et al. Consensus statement by The American Association of Clinical Endocrinologists and American College of Endocrinology on thc comprehensive type 2 diabetes management algorithm – 2018 executive summary. Endocr Pract. 2018;24(5):499.

Chapter 6
Cardiovascular Outcome Profiles of Anti-Diabetes Medications

Rekha B. Kumar

Case Presentation

A 71-year-old male with a 15-year history of type II diabetes and coronary artery disease who had one stent placed 3 years ago presents to his primary care doctor for management of obesity prior to knee replacement surgery. The patient is advised that he should lose approximately 25–30 lbs prior to undergoing surgery. His current BMI is 39 kg/m^2 with a height of 5′10 and weight of 270 lbs. He is on pioglitazone 45 mg and glimepiride 2 mg daily for his diabetes. He reports significant weight gain over the past decade, particularly after starting his current medicines. He tries to follow a 1700 kcal/day diet but finds that his blood sugar occasionally feels low although he is not checking his glucose frequently but eats granola bars when he feels this way. He often feels that his blood sugar drops overnight and needs to eat a snack at that time as well. His hemoglobin A1c is 8.3% and he has mild neuropathy.

R. B. Kumar (✉)
Comprehensive Weight Control Center, Division of Endocrinology, Diabetes and Metabolism, Weill Cornell Medical College, New York, NY, USA
e-mail: reb9037@med.cornell.edu

L. J. Aronne, R. B. Kumar (eds.), *Obesity Management*,
https://doi.org/10.1007/978-3-030-01039-3_6

Upon reviewing his medicines and diet history, his physician is concerned that his current regimen might be contributing to both weight gain and hypoglycemia, in turn exacerbating his obesity which is delaying his orthopedic procedure and further exacerbating his sedentary lifestyle. His vital signs are a BP of 135/85 and P of 65. His physical exam is significant for abdominal obesity with waist circumference of 45 inches and trace lower extremity edema bilaterally.

Assessment and Diagnosis

This patient has been referred for management of his obesity and diabetes perioperatively. Upon evaluation of his current diabetes regimen, it appears that his medicines are not optimized for weight control or his cardiac disease status. His sulfonylurea is likely causing intermittent hypoglycemia, leading him to eat more frequently, and his thiazolidinedione (pioglitazone) may be contributing to his lower extremity edema. In addition to these possible side effects, the patient's hemoglobin A1c is not optimized. He also has a history of coronary disease and would benefit from using diabetes medicine that also reduce cardiovascular mortality.

Management

In addition to focusing on avoiding weight gain and risk of hypoglycemia, the new standards of care set by the American Diabetes Association (ADA) in 2018 take into account current clinical trial data on cardiovascular outcomes. Consistent with the results of multiple cardiovascular outcome trials (CVOTs), new diabetes standards of treatment for adults with type II diabetes suggest that second-line therapy should include a medication that improves cardiovascular health after lifestyle modification and metformin therapy [1, 2]. The forest plot shows the reduction in major adverse cardiovascular events (MACE) in seven CVOTs on diabetes medications [3].

The patient is switched from pioglitazone 45 mg to metformin 500 mg twice daily which is titrated up to 1 g twice daily after 2 weeks. He is seen in the office 1 month later, and his glimepiride is stopped, and he is started on liraglutide 0.6 mg and told to titrate weekly up by 0.6 mg to reach 3 mg daily as tolerated. He is advised on a calorie-restricted, low-glycemic index diet.

Outcome

The patient is seen again 3 months later and is currently on metformin 1 mg twice daily and liraglutide 3 mg daily. He has lost 16 lbs, has improved control over his appetite, and is not waking up to eat overnight. His lower extremity edema is improved. His current HbA1c is 7.5% and has been cleared to have his knee replacement surgery.

Clinical Pearls and Pitfalls

- Patients' weight status and the presence of cardiovascular disease should be considerations when choosing medicines for diabetes.
- Recognize medication-induced weight gain in the context of medicines prescribed for type II diabetes.
- Correlate diet history with side effects of medicines that may be causing hypoglycemia and compensatory overeating.
- Be familiar with the diabetes medicines that have shown positive results in cardiovascular outcomes trials (CVOTs).

References

1. Rita R. Kalyani et al. ADA's Professional Practice Committee. Summary of revisions: standards of medical care in diabetes—2018. Diabetes Care. 2018;41(Supplement 1):S4–6.

2. Cefalo W, et al. Cardiovascular outcomes trials in type 2 diabetes: where do we go from here? Reflections from a diabetes care editors' expert forum. Diabetes Care. 2018;41(1):14–31.
3. Singh AK, Singh R. Recent cardiovascular outcome trials of antidiabetic drugs: a comparative analysis. Indian J Endocrinol Metab. 2017;21(1):4–10.

Part IV
Psychiatric Medication-Induced Weight Gain

Chapter 7
Selective Serotonin Reuptake Inhibitors (SSRIs) and Weight Gain

Leon I. Igel

Case Presentation

A 22-year-old female college student presents for a new patient visit. She has a history of depression and class 1 obesity (height 64 in, weight 186 lb, BMI 31.9 kg/m^2). The patient reports being diagnosed with depression by her prior internist, who initiated treatment with paroxetine 2 years ago. Her current dose of paroxetine is 40 mg daily. She feels that the paroxetine has improved her mood. However, she does note that since initiating the medication, she has gained 11 lb and has also experienced sexual side effects, including decreased libido. These side effects have contributed to some emotional and relationship distress. She maintains a healthy diet and exercises four to five times per week for 45–60 min per session. Despite

L. I. Igel (✉)
Comprehensive Weight Control Center, Division of Endocrinology, Diabetes and Metabolism, Weill Cornell Medical College, New York, NY, USA
e-mail: lei9004@med.cornell.edu

L. J. Aronne, R. B. Kumar (eds.), *Obesity Management*,
https://doi.org/10.1007/978-3-030-01039-3_7

these efforts, she has struggled to limit further weight gain. She would like to lose weight and asks for your help with respect to weight management.

Diagnosis and Assessment

This patient has a history of depression and reports a temporal association between initiation of paroxetine and her weight gain. For patients with psychiatric conditions, weight gain is a common complaint and often multifactorial. The antidepressant medications used for treatment frequently contribute to weight gain and/or make weight loss more difficult to achieve [1]. Among the numerous antidepressants, there is a broad range of weight gain potential, typically influenced by the duration of therapy [2]. Early weight gain after initiation of therapy is a strong predictor of long-term weight change [3]. Within the SSRI and tricyclic antidepressant (TCA) classes of drugs, paroxetine and amitriptyline, respectively, are associated with the greatest risk for weight gain [4, 5]. Lithium, mirtazapine, and the monoamine oxidase inhibitors (MAOIs) are also associated with weight gain [6].

There are only a limited number of antidepressants that are not associated with weight gain. The SSRIs fluoxetine and sertraline have been associated with weight loss with short-term use and relative weight neutrality with long-term use [4, 7, 8]. Bupropion is the only antidepressant that has been shown to consistently promote weight loss [8, 9, 10, 11]. Bupropion is a norepinephrine and dopamine reuptake inhibitor approved for the treatment of depression and to assist with smoking cessation. It also has a low rate of sexual side effects as compared to the SSRIs [12]. Bupropion has been demonstrated to decrease body weight by suppressing appetite and reducing food cravings [10]. It was approved by the Food and Drug Administration (FDA) for chronic weight management in 2014 in combination with another medication, naltrexone, under the brand name Contrave.

Management

Depending on the nature of the patient's depression, bupropion, fluoxetine, or sertraline might be reasonable alternatives to prevent or reduce paroxetine-induced weight gain.

As different classes of antidepressants are typically prescribed for different types of depression, the few agents that are weight neutral and weight-loss promoting are not appropriate for all patients with depression. For example, bupropion can be activating, so it could potentially exacerbate anxiety or be inappropriate for a patient with bipolar disorder. Thus, a patient with concomitant depression and anxiety might be a better candidate for a different antidepressant, which could lead to some weight gain but would better manage the individual's symptoms. In such cases, the rule of thumb would be to prescribe the lowest dose required for clinical efficacy for the shortest duration necessary. Significant early weight gain should prompt physicians to consider other therapeutic options and/or to initiate additional weight-controlling strategies [13]. The choice of antidepressant must ultimately be guided by best practice for the individual patient's circumstance [2, 14].

Outcome

The patient was initially cross-titrated from paroxetine to fluoxetine. Although she was able to lose most (8 lb) of the weight that she gained while on paroxetine, and her mood remained stable, the sexual side effects persisted. She was subsequently changed from fluoxetine to bupropion, which led to further weight loss. Six months after changing to bupropion, her weight stabilized at 168 lb (7 lb below her pre-paroxetine weight), with good mood control and without any unwanted sexual side effects. She has remained on bupropion XL 300 mg daily as a monotherapy, and it has been well tolerated.

Clinical Pearls and Pitfalls

- Always complete a thorough review of a patient's prescription and over-the-counter medicines to evaluate the possibility of medication-induced weight gain.
- Understand the weight profiles of various antidepressants (Table 7.1).
- Document the temporal relationship of medicines known to affect weight as part of a patient's weight gain history.
- Work in tandem with a patient's psychiatrist to treat depression and obesity concomitantly, if possible.
- If the only antidepressants that are effective for mood control also promote weight gain, reevaluate the medication dose, and confirm that the lowest doses required to control depression are being used.

TABLE 7.1 Psychiatric medications associated with weight gain, weight neutrality, and weight loss [14]

	Weight gain	Weight neutral/less weight gain	Weight loss
Antidepressants	Lithium MAOIs Mirtazapine SNRIs SSRIs (paroxetine) Tricyclic antidepressants (amitriptyline, doxepin, imipramine, nortriptyline)	SSRIs (fluoxetine, sertraline)	Bupropion
Antipsychotics	Clozapine Olanzapine Quetiapine Risperidone	Aripiprazole Lurasidone Ziprasidone	
Antiepileptics	Carbamazepine Gabapentin Pregabalin Valproic acid	Lamotrigine Levetiracetam Phenytoin	Topiramate Zonisamide

MAOI monoamine oxidase inhibitor; *SNRI* serotonin-norepinephrine reuptake inhibitors; *SSRI* selective serotonin reuptake inhibitor
Adapted from Igel et al. [14]

References

1. Apovian CM, Aronne L, Powell AG. Clinical management of obesity. West Islip: Professional Communications, Inc.; 2015.
2. Saunders KH, Igel LI, Shukla AP, et al. Drug-induced weight gain: rethinking our choices. J Fam Pract. 2016;65(11):780–782,784–786,788.
3. Vandenberghe F, Gholam-Rezaee M, Saigí-Morgui N, et al. Importance of early weight changes to predict long-term weight gain during psychotropic drug treatment. J Clin Psychiatry. 2015;76(11):e1417–23.
4. Serretti A, Mandelli L. Antidepressants and body weight: a comprehensive review and meta-analysis. J Clin Psychiatry. 2010;71(10):1259–72.
5. Rosenzweig-Lipson S, Beyer CE, Hughes ZA, et al. Differentiating antidepressants of the future: efficacy and safety. Pharmacol Ther. 2007;113(1):134–53.
6. Bray GA, Bouchard C. Chapter 17 – Drugs that cause weight gain and clinical alternatives to their use. In: Handbook of obesity – volume 2: clinical applications. 4th ed. Boca Raton: CRC Press; 2014. p. 220–9.
7. Norris SL, Zhang X, Avenell A, et al. Pharmacotherapy for weight loss in adults with type 2 diabetes mellitus. Cochrane Database Syst Rev. 2005;1:CD004096.
8. Domecq JP, Prutsky G, Leppin A, et al. Clinical review: drugs commonly associated with weight change: a systematic review and meta-analysis. J Clin Endocrinol Metab. 2015;100(2):363–70.
9. Gadde KM, Parker CB, Maner LG, Wagner HR, Logue EJ, Drezner MK, Krishnan KR. Bupropion for weight loss: an investigation of efficacy and tolerability in overweight and obese women. Obes Res. 2001;9:544–51.
10. Gadde KM, Xiong GL. Bupropion for weight reduction. Expert Rev Neurother. 2007;7(1):17–24.
11. Arterburn D, Sofer T, Boudreau DM, et al. Long-term weight change after initiating second-generation antidepressants. J Clin Forensic Med. 2016;5(4). pii: E48.
12. Patel K, Allen S, Haque MN, et al. Bupropion: a systematic review and meta-analysis of effectiveness as an antidepressant. Ther Adv Psychopharmacol. 2016 Apr;6(2):99–144.
13. American Diabetes Association, American Psychiatric Association, American Association of Clinical Endocrinologists, et al. Consensus development conference on antipsychotic drugs and obesity and diabetes. Diabetes Care. 2004;27(2):596–601.
14. Igel LI, Kumar RB, Saunders KH, Aronne LJ. Practical use of pharmacotherapy for obesity. Gastroenterology. 2017. pii: S0016–5085(17)30142–7.

Chapter 8
Antipsychotic Medication-Induced Weight Gain

Leon I. Igel

Case Presentation

A 35-year-old man is referred to you by his psychiatrist for assistance with weight management. The patient has a history of class 2 obesity (height 70 in, weight 258 lb, BMI 37 kg/m^2) and bipolar disorder managed with olanzapine. The olanzapine was started 1 year ago after SSRIs and SNRIs proved ineffective. While olanzapine has been helpful with respect to mood, the patient has gained 19 lb since initiating therapy. The patient's psychiatrist is hopeful that, together, you can formulate a plan to address the patient's weight while maintaining mood stability.

Diagnosis and Assessment

Individuals with psychiatric illnesses are at an increased risk of developing metabolic derangements due to multiple fac-

L. I. Igel (✉)
Comprehensive Weight Control Center, Division of Endocrinology, Diabetes and Metabolism, Weill Cornell Medical College, New York, NY, USA
e-mail: lei9004@med.cornell.edu

L. J. Aronne, R. B. Kumar (eds.), *Obesity Management*,
https://doi.org/10.1007/978-3-030-01039-3_8

tors, including the medications they require for treatment. This patient has experienced antipsychotic medication-induced weight gain. Because the patient has a diagnosis of bipolar disorder, bupropion may not be the best option for management as it has the potential to be activating. The patient did not experience sufficient improvement in mood with use of SSRIs or SNRIs. This patient has responded well to the antipsychotic olanzapine but unfortunately has experienced weight gain as a side effect. With respect to the antipsychotics, there are few weight-neutral options. Even the options that appear relatively weight neutral in short clinical trials demonstrate substantial variability in terms of a patient's individual weight change, especially with longer-term use. Lurasidone and ziprasidone appear to be the most weight neutral in the class [1–4], with aripiprazole generally demonstrating a lower risk for weight gain as well [5–7]. Olanzapine, clozapine, quetiapine, and risperidone are consistently associated with weight gain [8, 9], and studies demonstrate that patients may lose weight and develop improved glucose tolerance when switched from olanzapine to ziprasidone [10]. The antipsychotics appear to impact weight by multiple mechanisms, including effects on central appetite, satiety, and energy homeostasis pathways via alteration of dopaminergic, serotonergic, and histaminergic neurotransmission [11–13]. Secondary hyperprolactinemia caused by dopamine receptor antagonism may also dysregulate the hypothalamic-pituitary-adrenal axis and decrease insulin sensitivity [14]. Additional effects on endocannabinoid receptors, several neuropeptides, hormones, and cytokines appear to play a role [13, 15, 16].

Management

It is rarely possible to replace the mood-stabilizing effects of an antipsychotic medication with a different class of medication. However, combining an antipsychotic with another class of medication can often help to reduce the dose of antipsychotic required for treatment. Antiepileptics are frequently combined with antipsychotics in this manner. Antiepileptic agents have broad-ranging effects on weight, with some associated with substantial weight gain and others promoting weight loss. Valproic acid, gabapentin, pregabalin, and carbamazepine are associated with weight gain [17–19], while lamotrigine, levetiracetam, and phenytoin are considered relatively weight neutral [20]. Topiramate and zonisamide have been consistently associated with weight loss [15, 21]. In addition to anti-seizure activity, a subset of the antiepileptics are used off-label to treat psychiatric conditions, specifically bipolar disorder. Topiramate monotherapy is FDA approved for both the treatment of migraines and the management of seizures and is used off-label as a mood stabilizer in patients with bipolar disorder. Topiramate was approved by the FDA for chronic weight management in 2012 in combination with another medication, phentermine, under the brand name Qsymia.

Metformin may also help to mitigate weight gain associated with antipsychotic medication use [22–27]. Metformin is FDA approved for the treatment of type 2 diabetes mellitus (T2DM), but is commonly used off-label for other conditions including T2DM prevention in patients with prediabetes or impaired fasting glucose, treatment of polycystic ovarian syndrome (PCOS), and obesity/overweight (especially in patients with drug-induced weight gain). Since metformin appears to be a reasonably safe and effective adjunct to address antipsychotic-induced weight gain and metabolic abnormalities, this is a common prescription in this author's armamentarium.

When possible, practitioners should utilize weight-neutral or weight loss-promoting medications in the treatment of psychiatric conditions. If this is not feasible, weight gain can be prevented or lessened by selecting the lowest dose required to produce clinical efficacy for the shortest duration necessary. The addition of dedicated anti-obesity medications (liraglutide 3.0 mg (Saxenda), phentermine/topiramate ER (Qsymia), lorcaserin (Belviq) or naltrexone/bupropion ER (Contrave)) could be considered on a case-by-case basis, as directed by an obesity medicine specialist. Lifestyle modification, including diet and exercise counseling, is the cornerstone of treatment for obesity management and should be encouraged in tandem with all pharmacological treatment approaches, especially when a patient requires medication that can cause weight gain.

Outcomes

In collaboration with the patient's psychiatrist, the patient was cross-titrated from olanzapine to lurasidone with modest weight loss (6 lb), but the patient subsequently noticed sub-optimal mood control. Topiramate was then added with improved mood control and further weight loss (an additional 9 lb). To further enhance weight loss and offset antipsychotic-induced weight gain, metformin XR 500 mg twice daily was added with additional weight loss (8 lb) and unchanged mood control. The patient's weight stabilized below his pre-olanzapine baseline with excellent mood control on this combination.

Clinical Pearls and Pitfalls

- Antipsychotics impact weight via multiple mechanisms, including effects on central appetite, satiety, and energy homeostasis pathways via alteration of dopaminergic, serotonergic, and histaminergic neurotransmission and inducing insulin resistance.
- Patients should be aware of the possibility of weight gain on these medicines, and adherence to a balanced diet and exercise routine should be encouraged.
- An obesity medicine specialist should communicate with a patient's psychiatrist when treating antipsychotic-induced weight gain if alternative medicines are being suggested, or additional medicines are being prescribed to counteract the weight-gaining effects of the antipsychotic.
- The medicines that may safely mitigate this effect should be known to the obesity medicine specialists.

References

1. Leucht S, Cipriani A, Spineli L, et al. Comparative efficacy and tolerability of 15 antipsychotic drugs in schizophrenia: a multiple-treatments meta-analysis. Lancet. 2013 Sep 14;382(9896):951–62.
2. Simpson GM, Glick ID, Weiden PJ, et al. Randomized, controlled, double-blind multicenter comparison of the efficacy and tolerability of ziprasidone and olanzapine in acutely ill inpatients with schizophrenia or schizoaffective disorder. Am J Psychiatry. 2004;161:1837–47.
3. Komossa K, Rummel-Kluge C, Hunger H, et al. Ziprasidone versus other atypical antipsychotics for schizophrenia. Cochrane Database Syst Rev. 2009;4:CD006627.
4. Meyer JM, Mao Y, Pikalov A, et al. Weight change during long-term treatment with lurasidone: pooled analysis of studies in patients with schizophrenia. Int Clin Psychopharmacol. 2015 Nov;30(6):342–50.
5. Musil R, Obermeier M, Russ P, et al. Weight gain and antipsychotics: a drug safety review. Expert Opin Drug Saf. 2015 Jan;14(1):73–96.
6. Maayan L, Correll CU. Weight gain and metabolic risks associated with antipsychotic medications in children and adolescents. J Child Adolesc Psychopharmacol. 2011;21:517–35.
7. Hasnain M, Vieweg WV, Hollett B. Weight gain and glucose dysregulation with second-generation antipsychotics and antidepressants: a review for primary care physicians. Postgrad Med. 2012 Jul;124(4):154–67.
8. Lieberman JA, Stroup TS, McEvoy JP, et al. Effectiveness of antipsychotic drugs in patients with chronic schizophrenia. N Engl J Med. 2005;353:1209–23.
9. Fiedorowicz JG, Miller DD, Bishop JR, et al. Systematic review and meta-analysis of pharmacological interventions for weight gain from antipsychotics and mood stabilizers. Curr Psychiatr Rev. 2012;8(1):25–36.
10. Allison DB, Casey DE. Antipsychotic-induced weight gain: a review of the literature. J Clin Psychiatry. 2001;62(suppl 7):22–31.
11. He M, Deng C, Huang XF. The role of hypothalamic H1 receptor antagonism in antipsychotic-induced weight gain. CNS Drugs. 2013;27(6):423–34.
12. Ratliff JC, Barber JA, Palmese LB, et al. Association of prescription H1 antihistamine use with obesity: results from the National

Health and Nutrition Examination Survey. Obesity (Silver Spring). 2010;18:2398–400.
13. Himmerich H, Minkwitz J, Kirkby KC. Weight gain and metabolic changes during treatment with antipsychotics and antidepressants. Endocr Metab Immune Disord Drug Targets. 2015;15(4):252–60.
14. Baptista T. Body weight gain induced by antipsychotic drugs: mechanisms and management. Acta Psychiatr Scand. 1999;100(1):3–16.
15. Domecq JP, Prutsky G, Leppin A, et al. Clinical review: drugs commonly associated with weight change: a systematic review and meta-analysis. J Clin Endocrinol Metab. 2015;100(2):363–70.
16. Hasnain M, Vieweg WVR, Fredrickson SK. Metformin for atypical antipsychotic-induced weight gain and glucose metabolism dysregulation: review of the literature and clinical suggestions—ProQuest. CNS Drugs. 2010;24(3):193–206.
17. Verrotti A, D'Egidio C, Mohn A, et al. Weight gain following treatment with valproic acid: pathogenetic mechanisms and clinical implications. Obes Rev. 2011;12:e32–43.
18. DeToledo JC, Toledo C, DeCerce J, et al. Changes in body weight with chronic, high-dose gabapentin therapy. Ther Drug Monit. 1997;19:394–6.
19. Gaspari CN, Guerreiro CA. Modification in body weight associated with antiepileptic drugs. Arq Neuropsiquiatr. 2010;68:277–81.
20. Ben-Menachem E. Weight issues for people with epilepsy – a review. Epilepsia. 2007;48(Suppl 9):42–5.
21. Antel J, Hebebrand J. Weight-reducing side effects of the antiepileptic agents topiramate and zonisamide. Handb Exp Pharmacol. 2012;209:433–66.
22. Igel LI, Sinha A, Saunders KH, Apovian CM, Vojta D, Aronne LJ. Metformin: an old therapy that deserves a new indication for the treatment of obesity. Curr Atheroscler Rep. 2016;18(4):16.
23. Jesus C, Jesus I, Agius M. A review of the evidence for the use of metformin in the treatment of metabolic syndrome caused by antipsychotics. Psychiatr Danub. 2015;27(Suppl 1):S489–91.
24. Wu R-R, Zhao J-P, Guo X-F, et al. Metformin addition attenuates olanzapine-induced weight gain in drug-naive first-episode schizophrenia patients: a double-blind, placebo-controlled study. Am J Psychiatry. 2008;165(3):352–8.
25. Wu R-R, Zhao J-P, Jin H, et al. Lifestyle intervention and metformin for treatment of antipsychotic-induced weight gain: a randomized controlled trial. JAMA. 2008;299(2):185–93.

26. Jarskog LF, Hamer RM, Catellier DJ, et al. Metformin for weight loss and metabolic control in overweight outpatients with schizophrenia and schizoaffective disorder. Am J Psychiatry. 2013;170(9):1032–40.
27. Björkhem-Bergman L, Asplund AB, Lindh JD. Metformin for weight reduction in non-diabetic patients on antipsychotic drugs: a systematic review and meta-analysis. J Psychopharmacol. 2011;25(3):299–305.

Part V
Behavioral Interventions

Chapter 9
Nutritional Approaches and Self-Monitoring

Janet Feinstein

Case Presentation

A 55-year-old male with obesity presents to his obesity medicine specialist for weight management. His BMI is 41.92 kg/m^2, and he suffers from prediabetes, obstructive sleep apnea (OSA), hyperlipidemia, fatty liver, and gout. His medicines are atorvastatin 40 mg, allopurinol 300 mg, and vitamin D supplements.

He has previously lost weight by his own restrictive eating and with increased exercise. His most recent diet attempt resulted in a 25 lbs weight loss, but he began to experience increased hunger and subsequently started regaining weight the way he has in the past. He reports that he is now at his highest weight.

At his initial visit: BP 145/90, waist circumference 53″, Wt. 309 lbs. (140.2 kg).

Labs: HbA1c 5.9, TC 263, HDL 38, TG 233, LDL 178, TSH 4.2, Ast 36, Alt 54, vitamin B12 334, vitamin D 8, and CBC normal.

J. Feinstein (✉)
Comprehensive Weight Control Center, Division of Endocrinology, Diabetes and Metabolism, Weill Cornell Medical College, New York, NY, USA
e-mail: jlf2008@med.cornell.edu

L. J. Aronne, R. B. Kumar (eds.), *Obesity Management*,
https://doi.org/10.1007/978-3-030-01039-3_9

He is frustrated by his inability to maintain his weight loss with his own diet and exercise thus prompting him to seek treatment at a medically supervised weight management center. He expresses fear that if he cannot stick to a diet, he will need bariatric surgery which he does not want. He seeks advice on how to stick to a diet long term without regaining weight.

Assessment and Diagnosis

The patient suffers from class 3 obesity (BMI 40–44.9 kg/m^2) with several weight-related comorbidities.

Initial goal is to achieve a 5–10% weight loss due to health benefits seen even with mild reduction in body weight. This should be communicated to a patient to present them with manageable goals even if a much higher degree of weight loss is desired long term. A weight loss of 5–10% can improve health and well-being of individuals. Reduction in cardiovascular disease risk, blood pressure, blood glucose, arthritis, as well as mood and energy levels can be improved with this degree of weight reduction [1].

A comprehensive program of lifestyle modification is considered the first option for achieving this goal. Behavioral interventions for weight loss refer to a set of principles and techniques for helping individuals modify eating and thinking habits and activity that contribute to their excess weight.

Key features include self-monitoring, goal setting, nutrition, exercise, stimulus control, problem-solving, cognitive restructuring, and relapse prevention.

Self-monitoring refers to the observing and recording of eating, drinking, and physical activity patterns, followed by feedback on behaviors. Tracking can help patients increase their awareness of why and when they eat. They may learn they eat late at night or when they are lonely, bored, or depressed.

New technologies, including smartphones, diet tracking apps, wearable exercise trackers, and Wi-Fi-enabled scales (which automatically transmit weights from scale to server), all make it easier to monitor ones food intake, physical activity, and weight. The benefits of tracking include having data on dietary consumption as it is related to calorie and other nutrition goals. It allows reflection and planning food choices and introduces restraint and positive thinking and planning.

Often, patients are unaware of how many calories they are consuming, but when using an online food tracking app, they are able to ascertain their intake of calories and learn to make healthier choices through nutrition education, label reading, and portion control. Although it may vary, a calorie deficit of 500–700 calories/day is generally encouraged to promote a 1–2 lb. weight loss per week. The Mifflin equation is most accurate when estimating RMR (resting metabolic rate) [2] and helps form the basis for determining calorie needs.

While reducing calories is the most important component of achieving weight loss, physical activity plays a significant role, especially when maintaining weight loss [3].

During patient's initial visit, a detailed diet history is performed by the Registered Dietitian Nutritionist (RDN). This includes looking at a patient's usual pattern of eating, problem areas, and nutrient intake as well one's physical activity level. The RDN helps the patient become aware of his habits. Goal setting and key strategies for achieving those goals are discussed. SMART goals (Table 9.1) are very specific as they spell out what an individual will do, when, where, how, and for how long with the end goal being a lasting behavior change [4, 5].

TABLE 9.1 Defining SMART goals [4, 5]

Specific (have patient make a simple/directed goal)
Measurable (have this goal have attainable endpoints that can be assessed)
Achievable (patient and provider should agree this goal is realistic)
Relevant (realistic and pertains to the key issue)
Time bound (time limited and time sensitive)

There is no one diet prescription that works for all. While weight loss is essentially contingent on reducing total caloric intake, the composition of protein, fat, and carbohydrates in the diet (macronutrients) [6] is also important if the patient has underlying health issues. Since the patient in this case study has prediabetes, he was encouraged to follow a low-glycemic diet to help lower his blood glucose and insulin levels. For these patients, slow-digesting carbohydrates (vegetables, fruits, dairy, legumes, and small amounts of whole grains) are encouraged along with avoiding refined starches and sweets.

Initially we advise pairing protein-rich foods (leans meats, dairy, and legumes) at meals and snacks with healthy fat and fiber-rich vegetables. We encourage increasing fluid-rich foods (soups, salads, and unlimited non-starchy veggies) to help increase satiety. Small amounts of whole-grain starches are eaten at the end of the meal if needed.

Management

Patient was started on a low-glycemic eating regimen. His caloric goal was initially set at 1800–2000 calories per day. He started tracking on an online food tracker. He shared his weekly food and exercise diaries with the registered dietitian.

One of his goals was to start eating more vegetables at lunch. He also started preparing foods in advance rather than wait until meal time, thus removing the temptation to make the easy, unhealthy choice.

At his initial visit, patient was prescribed Metformin XR 500 mg per day, and then after 2 weeks, it was increased to twice daily. This medication is used off-label to treat prediabetes and can control hunger and cravings, while patients restrict their intake. Metformin used off label and pairing can reduce the progression of prediabetes to diabetes by 30% (Diabetes Prevention Program Study) [7]. Using anti-obesity pharmacotherapy can improve adherence to behavioral change and help promote long-term weight maintenance [8]. Many patients report they are able to adhere to their diet regimen longer since they are not feeling deprived because they are less hungry or have less cravings.

Patients are encouraged to become more active, first by increasing daily lifestyle exercise and then aiming for 150 min/week. Small bouts of exercise (10–15 min/time) are recommended for the inactive patient who finds exercise a challenge [9].

The patient started using a CPAP machine to help improve his sleep.

Initially, monthly visits are scheduled with a MD or RDN to help manage treatment, provide collaborative care and ongoing support. Once patients are stable and doing well, visits are encouraged every 2–3 months. Emphasis on changes in specific eating and activity behaviors are encouraged.

Outcome

Over the course of a year, the patient has lost 44 lbs. (14% of his total body weight). He continues to keep his food log; he reports at times he is less consistent but remains very aware of what he is eating. He knows if he exceeds 2200 calories/day in the absence of exercise, he will gain weight. Over the last several months, his weight has plateaued (Fig. 9.1).

He has hit some plateaus at certain times, especially when going through more stressful times. He has found a way to eat which has allowed him to break most of his bad habits and continues to receive nutrition and medical support to make him feel less hungry. He feels less tired and is more flexible. He realizes he doesn't need to be perfect, but the foundation of his eating is healthy. His weight loss has stayed off longer than any other previous diet attempts.

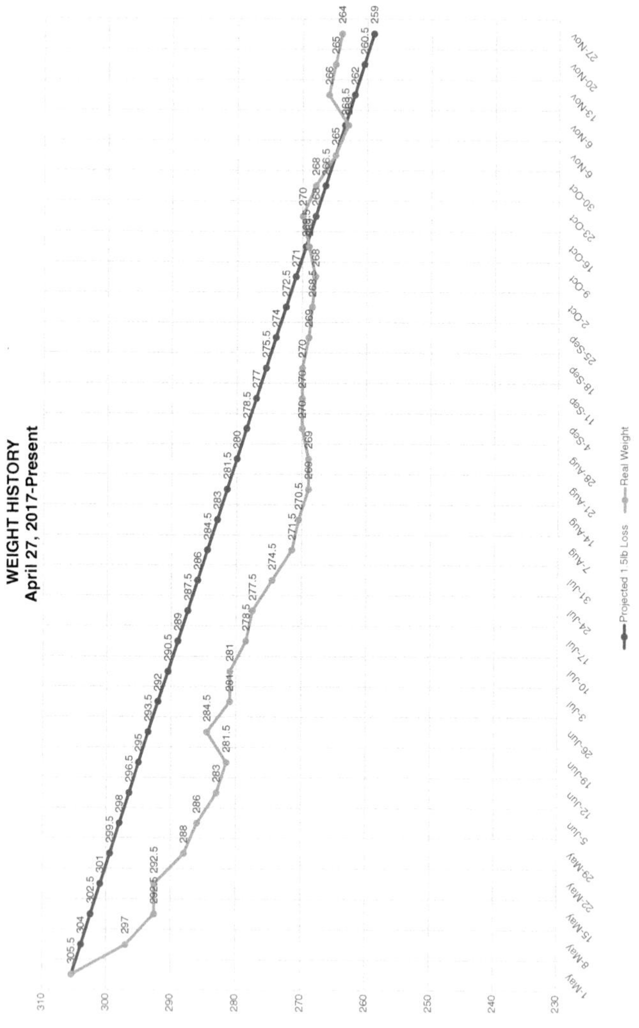

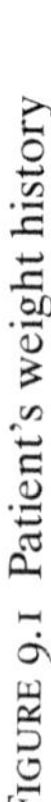

FIGURE 9.1 Patient's weight history

Clinical Pearls and Pitfalls

- Many patients do not know where to get the help they need to change their behaviors to help promote weight loss or achieve maintenance of weight loss.
- A registered dietitian can be an essential resource to providing information, support, and monitoring, while patients are on new diet plans. Tools used by RDNs are self-monitoring, goal setting, nutrition, exercise, stimulus control, problem-solving, cognitive restructuring, and relapse prevention.
- SMART goals are an example of a behavioral tool to achieve success.
- More collaborative care is needed between primary care physicians and patients and support between obesity care specialists.

References

1. Wing RR, Lang W, Wadden TA, et al. Benefits of modest weight loss in improving cardiovascular risk factors in overweight and obese individuals with type 2 diabetes. Diabetes Care. 2011;34:1481–6.
2. Frankenfield D, Yousey-Roth L, et al. Comparison of predictive equations for resting metabolic rate in healthy nonobese and obese adults: a systematic review. J Acad Nutr Diet. 2005;105:775–89.
3. American College of Sports Medicine. Appropriate physical activity intervention strategies for weight loss and prevention of weight gain for adults. Med Sci Sports Exerc. 2009;43:459–71.
4. Bovend'Eerdt TJ, Botell RE, Wade DT. Writing SMART rehabilitation goals and achieving attainment scaling: a practical guide. Clin Rehabil. 2009 Apr;23(4):352–61.
5. Perri MG, Nezu AM, McKelve WF, et al. Relapse prevention training and problem-solving therapy in the long-term management of obesity. J Consult Clin Psychol. 2001 Aug;69(4):722–6.
6. Saks FM, Bray GA, et al. Comparison of weight loss diets with different compositions of fat, protein and carbohydrates. N Engl J Med. 2009;360:859–73.

7. Knowler WC, Barrett-Connor E, et al. Diabetes prevention program research group reduction in incidence of type 2 diabetes with lifestyle intervention or metformin. N Engl J Med. 2002;346:393–403.
8. Apovian C, Aronne L, et al. Pharmacological management of obesity: an endocrine society clinical practice guideline. J Clin Endocrinol Metabolism. 2015;100(2):342–62.
9. Jensen MD, Ryan DH, Apovian CM, et al. AHA/ACC/TOS guideline for the management of overweight and obesity in adults: a report of the American College of Cardiology/American Heart Association task force on practical guidelines and the obesity society. J Am Coll Cardiol. 2014;63:2285–3023.

Chapter 10
Motivational Interviewing and Assessing Readiness to Change

Rachel Lustgarten

Case Presentation

A 47-year-old male presents to an obesity medicine specialist for weight management and is referred to a registered dietitian for guidance with his diet. His BMI is 34.4 kg/m^2 (247 lbs, 5′ 11″), and he suffers from depression, anxiety, hypertension, dyslipidemia, and GERD. The patient maintained a healthy weight throughout most of his early adult life. He played college tennis and exercised regularly as a young professional but has become more sedentary as his work hours have become more demanding and stressful. The patient is accompanied by his wife who is concerned about his increasing weight and health issues. His medicines are atorvastatin 40 mg for hypercholesterolemia, Prozac 20 mg for depression, lisinopril 20 mg for hypertension, Ambien 10 mg for insomnia, and Prilosec 20 mg for GERD. The patient states his refusal to add an additional medication for weight loss and

R. Lustgarten (✉)
Comprehensive Weight Control Center, Division of Endocrinology, Diabetes and Metabolism, Weill Cornell Medical College, New York, NY, USA
e-mail: ral2019@med.cornell.edu

L. J. Aronne, R. B. Kumar (eds.), *Obesity Management*,
https://doi.org/10.1007/978-3-030-01039-3_10

has no history of dietary modifications for weight control. His labs are normal, and his waist circumference is 48 inches.

Assessment and Diagnosis

The patient suffers from class 1 obesity (BMI 30–34.9 kg/m^2) with several weight-related comorbidities. The patient's affect is disinterested, and his wife, who made the appointment, answers many questions for him and interjects as he answers few questions. The patient states that he is not confident in his ability to make dietary changes and is not willing to give up his favorite foods. His diet recall reveals he skips breakfast and eats a large lunch and dinner meal via takeout or in a restaurant. Between meals and after dinner, the patient reports snacking on processed convenience foods high in calories, sugar, and fat if he is feeling stressed or cannot sleep. While he used to play tennis 3–5 times a week, he has not played in the past 2 years.

Implementation of a lifestyle and behavior modification program is indicated given the patient's BMI and comorbid conditions [1]. However, the patient's readiness to change (RTC) must first be assessed in order to tailor counseling in the most effective way. If the patient is not motivated for change or feels the barriers to change are too overwhelming, the clinician's intervention will be less impactful [2].

RTC can be qualified on the stages of change (SOC) continuum, precontemplation, contemplation, preparation, action, and maintenance, in which individuals move forward and at times backward, restarting the cycle [3]. Well-established self-report questionnaires such as the S-Weight and the P-Weight may be used in practice to assess patient's stages of change in weight management and behavior modification [2].

In the counseling session, the technique of motivational interviewing (MI) is often used as a tool to assess RTC and initiate behavior change. This patient-centered, collaborative approach can increase the patient's motivation and commitment to change [4]. Key components of MI include open-ended

TABLE 10.1 Examples of motivational interviewing questions

How is your current weight affecting your life right now?
What kinds of things have you done in the past to change your eating?
What strategies have worked for you in the past to increase physical activity?
How did you feel when you were engaging in regular physical activity?
What are your hopes for the future if you are able to become healthier?

question asked by practitioner (Table 10.1), a nonconfrontational style, and a concerted effort to minimize resistance. MI aims to enhance self-efficacy and personal control for behavior change. Originally used to treat addiction, MI is now used in many counseling settings in healthcare and can be of particular use in weight loss interventions [5].

In the initial session, the patient stated he was not confident in his ability to change certain dietary behaviors. When asked how he felt about adding a calorie-controlled breakfast meal, he identified with the contemplation stage of change as he knew skipping breakfast left him hungry, leading to overeating and poor food choices later in the day. He identified barriers to changing this behavior, including lack of time and access to healthy choices in the morning. Using the "ask-tell-ask" format of MI, the RDN inquired if the patient would be open to hearing some ideas for quick, easy, and healthy breakfasts [6]. The patient agreed, and the RDN shared the suggestion of using ready-to-drink protein meal replacements as a breakfast meal. The RDN then asked what the patient thought of that idea, and we met with acceptance. The patient expressed readiness to change his physical activity behaviors at this time, reflecting that he missed playing tennis and remembered it energized him during the day, reduced stress levels, and helped him sleep at night. The patient was guided toward creating SMART goals for his lifestyle modifications on his own without input from the RDN or his wife.

Management

After the initial consult, the patient restarted regular physical activity, playing single tennis, a moderate- to high-intensity exercise, three times per week at an indoor court near his home before work. He also added a protein meal replacement shake for breakfast daily. Monthly visits are scheduled with his RDN to offer continued support. After making initial changes, patient felt increased confidence and implemented self-monitoring strategies such as weighing in at home weekly. Sessions with the RDN continued to focus on RTC and used MI to assess readiness, importance, confidence, and barriers to change.

Outcome

In 1 year the patient has lost 28 lbs. (12%TBW). He remains in the maintenance stage of change with physical activity. He hit a weight loss plateau when he suffered an ankle sprain which resulted in his inability to play tennis and led to a relapse in change implementation. The patient enjoys autonomy over his dietary choices while communicating with his wife about how she can best support him in his weight loss journey. He eats less in response to stress and still consumes his favorite foods on occasion.

Clinical Pearls and Pitfalls

- Assessing motivation and RTC may be an essential step in identifying psychological obstacles or resistance toward lifestyle change in weight management patients and can lead to a more effective weight-control treatment intervention.
- RTC can be assessed via well-established questionnaires or verbally using MI.

- The motivational interviewing technique can be employed by members of the interdisciplinary care team to enhance weight loss in overweight and obese patients.
- A registered dietitian is a critical member of the obesity medicine care team, providing sound diet and activity prescriptions; however, solely providing educational counseling may not result in reduced body weight.
- A registered dietitian can be an essential resource in facilitating change talk providing support for patients to achieve autonomy in health behavior modification for weight loss and weight loss maintenance.

References

1. Jensen MD, Ryan DH, Apovian CM, et al. 2013 AHA/ACC/TOS guideline for the management of overweight and obesity in adults: a report of the American College of Cardiology/American Heart Association task force on practice guidelines and the Obesity Society. J Am Coll Cardiol. 2014;63(25 Pt B):2985–3023.
2. Ceccarini M, et al. Assessing motivation and readiness to change for weight management and control: an in-depth evaluation of three sets of instruments. Front Psychol. 2015;6:511.
3. Prochaska JO, Velicer WF. The transtheoretical model of health behavior change. Am J Health Promot. 1997;12:38–48.
4. DiLillo V, West DS. Motivational interviewing for weight loss. Psychiatr Clin North Am. 2011;34(4):861–9.
5. Resnicow K. Motivational interviewing: moving from why to how with autonomy support. Int J Behav Nutr Phys Act. 2012;9:19.
6. Shapiro J. Disclosure coaching: an ask-tell-ask model to support clinicians in disclosure conversations. J Patient Saf. 2018;16 [Epub ahead of print].

Part VI
Bariatric Surgery

Chapter 11
Surgical Options and Criteria for Bariatric Surgery

Beverly G. Tchang and Devika Umashanker

Case Presentation

A 41-year-old male presents for follow-up of weight management. He has struggled with obesity for most of his adult life and is currently at his highest weight of 300 lbs. He states that he cannot stop eating until he is "uncomfortably full" and sometimes eats because of stress and not necessarily hunger. In the past, he has successfully lost weight through commercial weight loss programs but has been unable to keep the weight off for more than 1 year. The most weight that he has ever lost was approximately 20 lbs. Because of his weight, he has difficulty walking and climbing stairs. He denies daytime somnolence, joint pain, exertional dyspnea, binge eating, or depressed mood. Past medical history is significant for hypertension, type 2 diabetes mellitus (T2DM), gastroesophageal

B. G. Tchang
Comprehensive Weight Control Center, Division of Endocrinology, Diabetes and Metabolism, Weill Cornell Medical College, New York, NY, USA

D. Umashanker (✉)
Department of Bariatric Surgery, Hartford Hospital, Hartford, CT, USA

L. J. Aronne, R. B. Kumar (eds.), *Obesity Management*,
https://doi.org/10.1007/978-3-030-01039-3_11

reflux disease (GERD), and dyslipidemia. His medications include hydrochlorothiazide 25 mg daily, atorvastatin 40 mg daily, metformin 500 mg daily, and omeprazole 40 mg daily. Physical exam is notable for a body mass index (BMI) of 43 kg/m^2 but is otherwise unremarkable. Labs reveal normal complete blood count, basic metabolic panel, and liver function tests. His fasting lipid panel is as follows: total cholesterol 184 mg/dL, LDL 97 mg/dL, HDL 30 mg/dL, and triglycerides 155 mg/dL; and his hemoglobin A1c is 7.4%. Today the patient inquires about his surgical options and would like to know if surgery is an option for him.

Assessment and Diagnosis

This patient has class 3 obesity (BMI $\geq$ 40 kg/m^2) with multiple weight-related comorbidities— hypertension, dyslipidemia, diabetes, and GERD—and is interested in losing weight. Bariatric surgery was previously considered a treatment option only for individuals who have "failed" medical/nutritional therapy, but because it has shown superior outcomes for long-term weight loss and resolution of comorbidities [1] in patients with severe obesity, it should be offered as an option in patients who continue to have obesity despite several attempts at weight loss.

As per the American Society for Metabolic and Bariatric Surgery (ASMBS) [2], indications for bariatric surgery are as follows:

- BMI $\geq$ 40 kg/m^2 or more than 100 pounds over ideal body weight.
- BMI $\geq$ 35 kg/m^2 and at least one or more obesity-related comorbidities such as T2DM, hypertension, sleep apnea and other respiratory disorders, nonalcoholic fatty liver disease, osteoarthritis, lipid abnormalities, gastrointestinal disorders, or heart disease.
- Inability to achieve a healthy weight loss sustained for a period of time with prior weight loss efforts.

This patient would qualify for bariatric surgery based on his BMI and presence of obesity-related comorbidities. Four bariatric procedures are currently performed in the United States (Table 11.1): adjustable gastric band (AGB), vertical sleeve gastrectomy (VSG), Roux-en-Y gastric bypass (RYGB), and biliopancreatic diversion-duodenal switch (BPD-DS). The choice of procedure depends on individual risk/benefit analysis.

Each bariatric procedure produces different amounts of total body weight loss, with VSG, RYGB, and BPD-DS resulting in more weight loss than AGB [3, 4] Bariatric surgery has also been shown to improve multiple comorbidities [5], resulting in decreased cardiovascular disease risk and overall mortality[6, 7]. Relevant to this patient, higher rates of T2DM remission were achieved with VSG, RYGB, and BPD-DS as compared to AGB [3]. This patient also has GERD, which may improve after RYGB [8] but has the potential to worsen after VSG. For these reasons, RYGB and BPD-DS would be acceptable options for this patient. However, because BPD-DS has the highest risk of micronutrient deficiency, postoperative complications, and mortality [9], RYGB would be the most appropriate choice for this patient.

Management

The patient underwent medical and psychological evaluation for bariatric surgery and was deemed an appropriate candidate for RYGB. He received nutritional counseling regarding the post-RYGB diet, with particular attention to potential vitamin deficiencies. He underwent RYGB with a subsequent uncomplicated postoperative course.

Outcome

Twelve months postoperatively, the patient has lost 35% of his initial body weight and has been able to discontinue his

TABLE 11.1 Comparisons of bariatric surgery types in the United States [5]

	Adjustable gastric band (AGB)	**Vertical sleeve gastrectomy (VSG)**	**Roux-en-Y gastric bypass (RYGB)**	**Biliopancreatic diversion-duodenal switch (BPD-DS)**
Description	An inflatable band is placed at the proximal stomach to create a small gastric pouch	About 80% of the stomach is removed to form a tubular structure	The stomach is resected to form a small gastric pouch, and then the small intestine is divided into two portions. The distal portion is connected to the pouch, resulting in bypass of the duodenum, and the proximal portion is reconnected to the jejunum.	The stomach is resected to form a vertical sleeve, and then the small intestine is divided into two portions. The distal portion is connected to the pylorus, and the proximal portion is reconnected to the jejunum such that about 75% of the small intestine is bypassed
	Restrictive	Restrictive	Restrictive and malabsorptive	Restrictive and malabsorptive

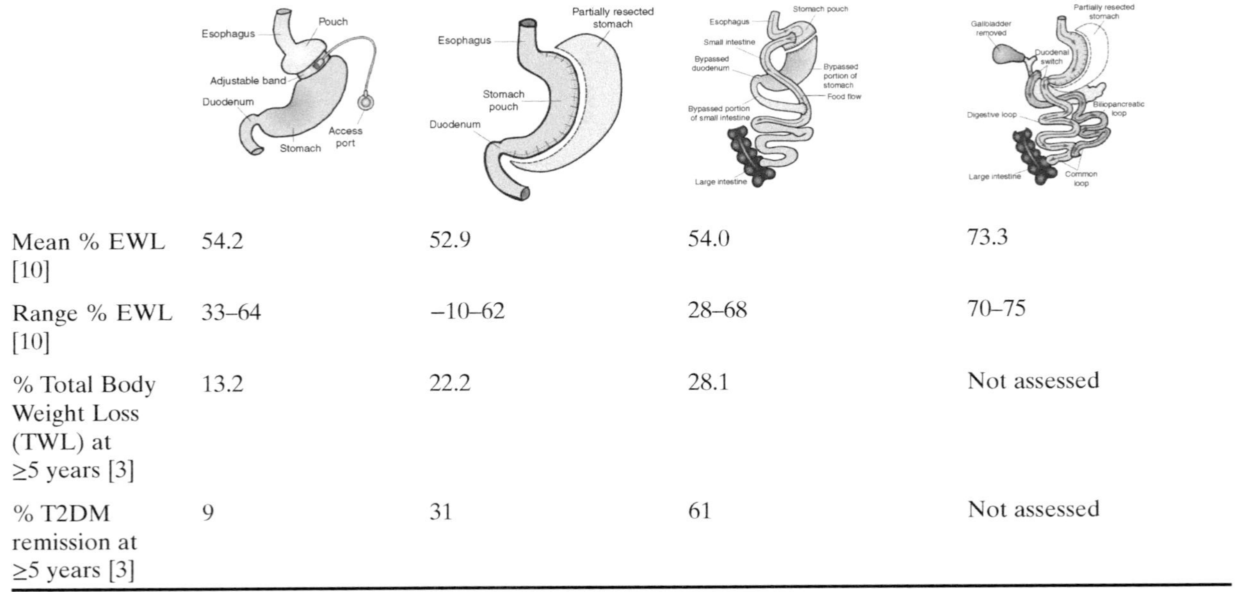

Mean % EWL [10]	54.2	52.9	54.0	73.3
Range % EWL [10]	33–64	−10–62	28–68	70–75
% Total Body Weight Loss (TWL) at ≥5 years [3]	13.2	22.2	28.1	Not assessed
% T2DM remission at ≥5 years [3]	9	31	61	Not assessed

(continued)

TABLE 11.1 (continued)

	Adjustable gastric band (AGB)	**Vertical sleeve gastrectomy (VSG)**	**Roux-en-Y gastric bypass (RYGB)**	**Biliopancreatic diversion-duodenal switch (BPD-DS)**
Advantages	Lowest risk of micronutrient deficiency Adjustable Reversible	Lower risk of micronutrient deficiency compared to RYGB Produces favorable changes of gut hormones to promote satiety and reduce hunger More effective at inducing sustained diabetes remission than AGB	Produces favorable changes of gut hormones to promote satiety and reduce hunger More effective at inducing sustained diabetes remission compared to VSG. Reversible	Produces favorable changes of gut hormones to promote satiety and reduce hunger. Most effective at inducing sustained diabetes remission Partially reversible
Disadvantages	Lowest efficacy and durability of all bariatric surgeries Highest rate of reoperation Risk of band erosion	Nonreversible Potential to exacerbate pre-existing GERD	Higher risk of micronutrient deficiency compared to VSG Potential to develop early or late dumping syndrome	Highest risk of micronutrient deficiency Highest postoperative complication rates and mortality risk

EWL excess weight loss
%TWL can be estimated from %EWL. %TWL is approximately one-half the numerical value of %EWL [5, 10]

hypertension and diabetes medications. Both his blood pressure and his hemoglobin A1c are at goal. He has been able to reduce his omeprazole dose by half.

Clinical Pearls and Pitfalls

- Individuals with BMI ≥ 40 kg/m^2 or BMI ≥ 35 kg/m^2 and at least one or more obesity-related comorbidities should be offered bariatric surgery.
- Bariatric surgery has been shown to improve comorbidities resulting in decreased cardiovascular disease risk and overall mortality.
- Selection of the appropriate bariatric procedure is individualized to each patient based on his/her comorbidities and risk/benefit assessment.

References

1. Picot J, et al. The clinical effectiveness and cost-effectiveness of bariatric (weight loss) surgery for obesity: a systematic review and economic evaluation. Health Technol Assess. 2009;13:1–190, 215–357.
2. American Society of Metabolic and Bariatric Surgery. Who is a candidate for bariatric surgery? 2018. https://asmbs.org/patients/who-is-a-candidate-for-bariatric-surgery.
3. Brethauer SA, et al. Can diabetes be surgically cured? Long-term metabolic effects of bariatric surgery in obese patients with type 2 diabetes mellitus. Ann Surg. 2013;258:628–36.
4. Courcoulas AP, et al. Longitudinal Assessment of Bariatric Surgery (LABS) Consortium. Weight change and health outcomes at 3 years after bariatric surgery among individuals with severe obesity. JAMA. 2013;310:2416–25.
5. Apovian CM, Aronne LJ, Powell AG. Clinical Management of Obesity Bariatric Surgery, 1st edition. West Islip: Professional Communications. 2015;10:251–85.
6. Sjostrom L. Review of the key results from the Swedish Obese Subjects (SOS) trial – a prospective controlled intervention study of bariatric surgery. J Intern Med. 2013;273(3):219–34.

7. Jensen MD, et al. 2013 AHA/ACC/TOS Guideline for the management of overweight and obesity in adults. A report of the American College of Cardiology/American Heart Association task force on practice guidelines and the obesity society. Circulation. 2014;129:S102–38.
8. Madalosso CA. The impact of gastric bypass on gastroesophageal reflux disease in morbidly obese patients. Ann Surg. 2016;263(1):110–6.
9. American Society of Metabolic and Bariatric Surgery. Bariatric surgery procedures. 2018. https://asmbs.org/patients/bariatric-surgery-procedures.
10. O'Brien PE, et al. Long-term outcomes after bariatric surgery: fifteen-year follow-up of adjustable gastric banding and a systematic review of the bariatric surgical literature. Ann Surg. 2013;257:87–94.

Chapter 12
Postoperative Management and Nutritional Deficiencies

Beverly G. Tchang

Case Presentation

A 52-year-old woman presents for her annual postoperative bariatric surgery appointment. She underwent Roux-en-Y gastric bypass (RYGB) 3 years ago. Since then, she has lost more than 100 lbs. and no longer requires antihypertensive medication. In reviewing her diet, she reports becoming a vegan over the past year and has continued to avoid sweets and carbonated beverages. Six months ago, she sustained a left wrist fracture after tripping on the sidewalk. She also reports generalized fatigue and tingling in her fingers and toes for the past 2 months. She admits to not taking her vitamins as recommended. On exam, she weighs 161 lbs. with a BMI of 26.8 kg/m^2. She is afebrile with a blood pressure of 120/60 and heart rate of 95 beats/min. A beefy, red tongue and pale conjunctiva are notable. The rest of her exam including neurological assessment is otherwise normal. Labs reveal

B. G. Tchang (✉)
Comprehensive Weight Control Center, Division of Endocrinology, Diabetes and Metabolism, Weill Cornell Medical College, New York, NY, USA
e-mail: bgt9001@med.cornell.edu

L. J. Aronne, R. B. Kumar (eds.), *Obesity Management*,
https://doi.org/10.1007/978-3-030-01039-3_12

hemoglobin 10.8 g/dl [normal 11.2–14.7] and hematocrit 33.7% [normal 33.8–43.3] with an MCV of 105 fL [normal 79.4–94.7]. Serum folate is 10 ng/ml [normal ≥4.8] and vitamin B12 is 150 pg/ml [normal 299–1054]. Methylmalonic acid is elevated. 25-hydroxyvitamin D is 8 ng/ml [normal ≥20 ng/ml]. Basic metabolic panel is normal and other micronutrient labs are normal.

Assessment and Diagnosis

All bariatric procedures carry a risk for micronutrient deficiency, which may be due to preoperative deficiencies, overly restrictive diets, the type of surgery, or postoperative emesis and food intolerance. Malabsorptive procedures such as RYGB and biliopancreatic diversion-duodenal switch (BPD-DS) confer a higher risk of micronutrient deficiency than purely restrictive procedures, like the adjustable gastric band, because food is rerouted to bypass portions of the small intestine (i.e., duodenum, proximal jejunum), which are vital sites of nutrient absorption [1]. Even the vertical sleeve gastrectomy carries a risk of micronutrient deficiency due to the increase in gastric transit time, resulting in less time for absorption [2]. Because of these risks, the American Society for Metabolic and Bariatric Surgery (ASMBS) recommends that all patients are evaluated prior to surgery for certain micronutrient deficiencies, placed on prophylactic supplementation postoperatively, and are screened regularly for new deficiencies since they can develop many years after the initial surgery [3]. See Table 12.1 for signs and symptoms of pertinent micronutrient deficiencies.

This patient is at high risk for micronutrient deficiency given her history of RYGB, nonadherence to vitamin supplementation, and restricted diet. RYGB is both a malabsorptive and restrictive procedure that allows food to bypass the duodenum and part of the jejunum. Post-RYGB, patients are placed on multivitamins to provide additional thiamine, zinc, copper, iron, folate, vitamin A, vitamin E, and vitamin K, as

Table 12.1 Signs and symptoms of micronutrient deficiencies

	Early signs/symptoms	Advanced signs/symptoms
Thiamine (B1)	Dry beriberi (without edema): Brisk tendon reflexes, peripheral neuropathy or polyneuritis (with or without paresthesias), muscle weakness or pain of upper and lower extremities, gait ataxia, convulsions Wet beriberi: Heart failure with high cardiac output, lower extremity edema, tachycardia or bradycardia, lactic acidosis, dyspnea, heart hypertrophy and dilation Other/gastroenterologic: Slow gastric emptying, nausea, vomiting, jejunal dilation or megacolon, constipation	Wernicke's encephalopathy: Polyneuropathy and ataxia, ophthalmoplegia or nystagmus, confabulation, short-term memory loss Wernicke-Korsakoff syndrome: Encephalopathy plus psychosis
Vitamin B12	Pernicious anemia/megaloblastic anemia, pale with slightly icteric skin and eyes, glossitis (magenta or "beefy red" tongue) Numbness and paresthesia (tingling or prickly feeling) in extremities, ataxia, tinnitus Light-headedness or vertigo, dyspnea, fatigue, anorexia, diarrhea, palpitations	Angina or symptoms of congestive failure Altered mental status, ranging from mild irritability and forgetfulness to severe dementia or frank psychosis
Folate	Megaloblastic anemia Changes in pigmentation or ulceration of skin, nails, or oral mucosa	

(continued)

Table 12.1 (continued)

	Early signs/symptoms	Advanced signs/symptoms
Iron	Microcytic anemia Spoon-shaped nails (koilonychias), vertical ridges on nails Fatigue, light-headedness, palpitations, dyspnea, glossitis, dysphagia, decreased immune function, enteropathy	
Calcium	Cramping, tetany, muscle weakness Hypocalcemia Osteoporosis or fractures	
Vitamin D	Hypocalcemia, tetany, tingling, cramping Metabolic bone disease, rachitic tetany	
Vitamin A	Nyctalopia (night blindness or difficulty seeing in dim light), Bitot's spots (foamy white spots on sclera of eye), endophthalmitis, poor wound healing Hyperkeratinization of the skin, loss of taste	Blindness, corneal damage, xerosis, keratomalacia, perforation
Vitamin E	Hyporeflexia, gait disturbances, neurologic damage, muscle weakness, decreased proprioception, and vibration Ophthalmoplegia, nystagmus, nyctalopia Hemolytic anemia	

Vitamin K	Hemorrhage due to deficiency of prothrombin and other factors Easy bruising, petechiae, bleeding gums, delayed blood clotting, heavy menses, epistaxis	Osteoporosis
Zinc	Rash, acne Hypogeusia or ageusia (change in or absence of taste) Immune deficiency, increased infections Infertility	Hypogonadism Alopecia, skin lesions/rashes (bullous pustular dermatitis, acrodermatitis enteropathica) Diarrhea, anorexia, night blindness, recurrent infections, delayed wound healing
Copper	Hypochromic anemia, neutropenia, pancytopenia Hypopigmentation of hair, skin, nails Hypercholesterolemia Impaired biomarkers of bone metabolism	Gait abnormalities

Adapted from ASMBS Guidelines [3]

well as separate vitamin B12, vitamin D, and calcium supplementation, with special considerations for premenopausal women [3]. Her vegan diet also limits her dietary intake of vitamin B12, iron, calcium, and zinc [4].

The patient's symptoms, exam findings, and labs are consistent with vitamin D deficiency and vitamin B12 deficiency causing a macrocytic anemia. The reported prevalence of vitamin D deficiency is 100% in bariatric surgery patients; in contrast, the prevalence of vitamin B12 deficiency is 20% at 2–5 years after RYGB [3].

Management

Per ASMBS, the recommended vitamin D3 dose is 3000 IU per day with a goal vitamin D level of >30 ng/ml. For vitamin B12 deficiency, oral repletion doses range from 350 to 500 mcg daily; a parenteral alternative is available as an intramuscular or subcutaneous injection if oral supplementation cannot overcome the problem of poor absorption. Oral vitamin B12 is a reasonable first attempt at supplementation if the deficiency is found on screening and the patient does not have significant signs or symptoms. However, because this patient is already experiencing hematologic and neurologic consequences, of which the latter is irreversible, she was started vitamin B12 intramuscular injections at 1000 mcg daily for 7 days and then monitored closely. The patient was also counseled on safely continuing a vegan diet.

Outcome

After 2 months of vitamin D 3000 IU daily, repeat labs showed a higher 25-hydroxyvitamin D level of 15 ng/ml, which is still in the deficient range. Dose adjustments were made, and the patient is now vitamin D replete on a maintenance dose of 50,000 IU once a week. Her vitamin B12 levels normalized after aggressive treatment, and she has continued to receive vitamin B12 injections of 1000 mcg once a month for maintenance. She continues to follow up annually to have her levels of vitamin D and vitamin B12 checked, as well as to continue surveillance for thiamine, folate, iron, vitamin A, zinc, and copper deficiencies.

Clinical Pearls and Pitfalls

- All bariatric surgeries carry some risk for micronutrient deficiencies, with malabsorptive procedures carrying a greater risk than purely restrictive procedures.
- Patients should be evaluated preoperatively and postoperatively on a regular basis to screen for micronutrient deficiencies.
- Management of micronutrient deficiencies often requires high doses of supplementation.

References

1. Basu TK, Donaldson D. Intestinal absorption in health and disease: micronutrients. Best Pract Res Clin Gastroenterol. 2003 Dec;17(6):957–79.
2. Apovian CM, Aronne LJ, Powell AG. Clinical Management of Obesity Bariatric Surgery, 1st edition. West Islip: Professional Communications. 2015;10:251–85.
3. Parrott J, et al. American Society for Metabolic and Bariatric Surgery Integrated Health Nutritional Guidelines for the surgical weight loss patient 2016 update: micronutrients. Surg Obes Relat Dis. 2017 May;13(5):727–41.
4. Craig WJ. Health effects of vegan diets. Am J Clin Nutr. 2009 May;89(5):1627S–1633S.g.

Part VII
Pharmacotherapy for Obesity

Chapter 13
Choosing a Medication

Katherine H. Saunders

Case Presentation

A 29-year-old woman presents to an obesity medicine specialist for weight management. Her body mass index (BMI) is 32 kg/m^2 (198 lbs, 5′6″), and she suffers from depression, irritable bowel syndrome with diarrhea (IBS-D), and migraines. Her medications are oral contraceptive pills, sertraline 150 mg daily, and sumatriptan 50 mg as needed for migraines, which occur two to four times per month. She has lost weight successfully several times in the past through diet and exercise; however, she always regains the weight. A few months ago, she started a low carbohydrate diet and an exercise routine. After losing 8 pounds (206 → 198 lbs), she quickly reached a weight plateau despite ongoing diet and exercise. She is very frustrated and does not understand why she is unable to lose weight and maintain weight loss. She denies history of anxiety or nephrolithiasis. Her exam is within normal limits, and her laboratory data reveal no

K. H. Saunders (✉)
Comprehensive Weight Control Center, Division of Endocrinology, Diabetes and Metabolism, Weill Cornell Medical College, New York, NY, USA
e-mail: kph2001@med.cornell.edu

L. J. Aronne, R. B. Kumar (eds.), *Obesity Management*,
https://doi.org/10.1007/978-3-030-01039-3_13

abnormalities besides low high density lipoprotein cholesterol (HDL-C), high low-density lipoprotein cholesterol (LDL-C), and elevated triglycerides.

Assessment and Diagnosis

This patient suffers from class I obesity (BMI 30–34.9 kg/m^2) complicated by hyperlipidemia, IBS-D, depression, and migraines. She has failed multiple trials of lifestyle modifications so she would be a good candidate for anti-obesity pharmacotherapy in addition to ongoing lifestyle interventions.

According to the 2013 American College of Cardiology/American Heart Association/The Obesity Society (AHA/ACC/TOS) Guideline for the Management of Overweight and Obesity in Adults, patients who are obese or overweight with cardiovascular risk factors should be counseled on diet, physical activity, and other lifestyle modifications [1]. Unfortunately behavioral interventions alone do not lead to sustained weight loss for many patients because adaptive physiologic responses reduce energy expenditure and increase appetite [2–4]. Studies demonstrate that subjects burn fewer calories with the same exercise and notice more hunger and cravings at a lower weight. This phenomenon, known as metabolic adaptation or counteracts weight loss and leads to weight regain.

Anti-obesity pharmacotherapy is one strategy to combat these changes in energy expenditure and appetite. Both the 2013 AHA/ACC/TOS Guideline for the Management of Overweight and Obesity in Adults and the Endocrine Society's 2015 clinical practice guidelines on pharmacological management of obesity recommend considering anti-obesity pharmacotherapy for patients with BMI $\geq$ 30 kg/m^2 or $\geq$ 27 kg/m^2 with weight-related comorbidities including type 2 diabetes, hypertension, dyslipidemia, and obstructive sleep apnea [1, 5]. The six most widely prescribed anti-obesity medications approved by the Food and Drug Administration (FDA) are phentermine, orlistat, phentermine/topiramate extended release (ER), lorcaserin, naltrexone sustained release (SR)/ bupropion SR, and liraglutide 3.0 mg (Table 13.1).

Most of the anti-obesity medications target the arcuate nucleus of the hypothalamus to stimulate anorexigenic pro-opiomelanocortin (POMC) neurons, which promote increased energy expenditure and satiety. As obesity is a chronic disease, all of the agents besides phentermine monotherapy (which was approved in 1959) are approved for long-term use. When an anti-obesity medication is discontinued, there may be some weight regain, similar to an increase in blood pressure when an antihypertensive agent is stopped.

It is necessary to discuss with patients that anti-obesity agents are only one component of a comprehensive weight management plan, which also includes diet, exercise, and lifestyle modifications. Anti-obesity pharmacotherapy can improve adherence to behavioral interventions in addition to many outcomes including weight-related quality of life, waist circumference, blood pressure, lipids, glucose, and hemoglobin A1c. As a result, it is often possible for an anti-obesity agent to replace one or more medications for weight-related comorbid conditions such as type 2 diabetes and hypertension.

Many patients will ask how much weight loss is sufficient. Research has shown that weight loss of 5–10% in patients who are obese or overweight can lead to a clinically significant reduction in cardiovascular disease risk. This modest weight loss can not only improve blood pressure, blood sugar, HDL, and triglycerides, but it can increase insulin sensitivity in muscle, liver, and adipose tissue [6, 7].

Before starting pharmacotherapy for obesity, it is important to ask two questions [8]:

1) Are there contraindications, drug-drug interactions, or undesirable adverse effects associated with this medication that could be problematic for the patient?
2) Can this medication improve other symptoms or conditions the patient has?

Table 13.1 Overview of anti-obesity medications

Medication	Mechanism, dosage, and available formulations	Trial and duration	Trial arms	Weight loss (%)	Most common adverse events	Good candidates	Poor candidates
Phentermine (*Adipex,*[1] *Ionamin,*[2] *Lomaira,*[3] *Suprenza*[4]) Schedule IV controlled substance NOTE: approved for short-term use	Adrenergic agonist 8 mg–37.5 mg daily Capsule, tablet	*Aronne LJ, et al.*[5] 28 weeks	15 mg daily 7.5 mg daily Placebo (topiramate ER and phentermine/ topiramate ER arms excluded)	6.06[a] 5.45[a] 1.71	Dry mouth, insomnia, dizziness, irritability	Younger patients who need assistance with appetite suppression	Patients with uncontrolled hypertension, active or unstable coronary disease, hyperthyroidism, glaucoma, anxiety, insomnia, or patients who are generally sensitive to stimulants; patients with a history of drug abuse or recent MAOI use; patients who are pregnant
Orlistat (*Alli,*[6] *Xenical*[7])	Lipase inhibitor 60–120 mg TID with meals Capsule	*XENDOS*[8] 208 weeks	120 mg TID Placebo	9.6 (week 52)[a] 5.25 (week 208)[a] 5.61 (week 52) 2.71 (week 208)	Fecal urgency, oily stool, flatus with discharge, fecal incontinence	Patients with hypercho-lesterolemia and/or constipation who can limit their intake of dietary fat	Patients with malabsorption syndromes, or other gastrointestinal conditions that predispose to GI upset/diarrhea; patients who cannot modify the fat content of their diets; patients who are pregnant

Phentermine/ topiramate extended release (Qsymia)[9] Schedule IV controlled substance	Adrenergic agonist/ neurostabilizer 3.75/23–15/92 mg daily (dose titration) Capsule	*EQUIP*[10] 56 weeks	15/92 mg daily	10.9[a]	Paresthesias, dizziness, dysgeusia, insomnia, constipation, dry mouth	Younger patients who need assistance with appetite suppression	Patients with uncontrolled hypertension, active or unstable coronary disease, hyperthyroidism, glaucoma, anxiety, insomnia, or patients who are generally sensitive to stimulants; patients with a history of drug abuse or recent MAOI use; patients with a history of nephrolithiasis; patients who are pregnant
			3.75/23 mg daily	5.1[a]			
			Placebo	1.6			
		CONQUER[11] 56 weeks	15/92 mg daily	9.8[a]			
			7.5/46 mg daily	7.8[a]			
			Placebo	1.2			
		SEQUEL[12] 108 weeks (52-week extension of CONQUER trial)	15/92 mg daily	10.5[a]			
			7.5/46 mg daily	9.3[a]			
			Placebo	1.8 (weeks 0–108)			

(continued)

Table 13.1 (continued)

Medication	Mechanism, dosage, and available formulations	Trial and duration	Trial arms	Weight loss (%)	Most common adverse events	Good candidates	Poor candidates
Lorcaserin (Belviq, Belviq XR)[13] Schedule IV controlled substance	Serotonin (5-HT)$_{2C}$ receptor agonist 10 mg BID or 20 mg XR daily Tablet	*BLOOM*[14] 52 weeks	10 mg BID Placebo	5.8[a] 2.2	Headache, dizziness, fatigue, nausea, dry mouth, constipation	Patients who report inadequate meal satiety	Patients on other serotonin-modulating medications and patients with known cardiac valvular disease; patients who are pregnant
		BLOSSOM[15] 52 weeks	10 mg BID 10 mg daily Placebo	5.8[a] 4.7[a] 2.8			
		BLOOM-DM[16] 52 weeks	10 mg BID 10 mg daily Placebo	4.5[a] 5.0[a] 1.5			

Naltrexone/ bupropion sustained-release (Contrave)[17]	Opioid receptor antagonist/ dopamine and norepinephrine reuptake inhibitor 8/90 mg daily to 16/180 mg BID Tablet	*COR-I*[18] 56 weeks	16/180 mg BID 8/180 mg BID Placebo	6.1[a] 5.0[a] 1.3		Nausea, vomiting, constipation, headache, dizziness, insomnia, dry mouth	Patients who describe cravings for food and/or addictive behaviors related to food; patients who are trying to quit smoking, reduce alcohol intake, and/ or have concomitant depression	Patients with uncontrolled hypertension, uncontrolled pain, recent MAOI use, history of seizures, or any condition that predisposes to seizure such as anorexia/ bulimia nervosa, abrupt discontinuation of alcohol, benzodiazepines, barbiturates, or antiepileptic drugs; patients who are pregnant
		COR-II[19] 56 weeks	16/180 mg BID Placebo	6.4[a] 1.2				
		COR-BMOD[20] 56 weeks	16/180 mg BID Placebo	9.3[a] 5.1				
		COR-DIABETES[21] 56 weeks	16/180 mg BID Placebo	5.0[a] 1.8				

(continued)

Table 13.1 (continued)

Medication	Mechanism, dosage, and available formulations	Trial and duration	Trial arms	Weight loss (%)	Most common adverse events	Good candidates	Poor candidates
Liraglutide 3.0 mg (Saxenda)[22]	GLP-1 receptor agonist 0.6–3.0 mg daily Prefilled pen for subcutaneous injection	*SCALE Obesity and Prediabetes*[23] 56 weeks	3.0 mg daily Placebo	8.0[a] 2.6	Nausea, vomiting, diarrhea, constipation, dyspepsia, abdominal pain	Patients who report inadequate meal satiety, and/or have type 2 diabetes, prediabetes, or impaired glucose tolerance; patients requiring use of concomitant psychiatric medications	Patients with an aversion to needles, history of pancreatitis, personal or family history of medullary thyroid carcinoma, or multiple endocrine neoplasia syndrome type 2; patients who are pregnant
		SCALE Diabetes[24] 56 weeks	3.0 mg daily 1.8 mg daily Placebo	6[a] 4.7[a] 2.0			
		SCALE Maintenance[25] 56 weeks (after initial ≥5% weight loss with LCD)	3.0 mg daily Placebo	6.2[a] 0.2			

BID twice daily, *GI* gastrointestinal, *GLP-1* Glucagon-like peptide-1, *LCD* low-calorie diet, *MAOI* monoamine oxidase inhibitor, *TID* three times daily, *XR* extended release

[a]$p < 0.001$ vs. placebo

Adapted from: Saunders et al. [8], Igel et al. [24], Saunders et al. [25]

[1]Adipex [package insert]. Tulsa, OK: Physicians Total Care, Inc.; 2012

[2]Ionamin [package insert]. Rochester, NY: Celltech Pharmaceuticals, Inc.; 2006
[3]Lomaira [package insert]. Newtown, PA: KVK-TECH, Inc.; 2016
[4]Suprenza [package insert]. Cranford, NJ: Akrimax Pharmaceuticals, LLC; 2013
[5]Aronne et al. [26]
[6]Alli [package insert]. Moon Township, PA: GlaxoSmithKline Consumer Healthcare, LP; 2015
[7]Xenical [package insert]. South San Francisco, CA: Genentech USA, Inc.; 2015
[8]Torgerson et al. [13]
[9]Qsymia [package insert]. Mountain View, CA: VIVUS, Inc.; 2012
[10]Allison et al. [10]
[11]Gadde et al. [11]
[12]Garvey et al. [12]
[13]Belviq [package insert]. Zofingen, Switzerland: Arena Pharmaceuticals; 2012
[14]Smith et al. [14]
[15]Fidler et al. [15]
[16]O'Neil et al. [16]
[17]Contrave [package insert]. Deerfield, IL: Takeda Pharmaceuticals America, Inc.; 2014
[18]Greenway et al. [17]
[19]Apovian et al. [18]
[20]Wadden et al. [19]
[21.]Hollander et al. [20]
[22.]Saxenda [package insert]. Plainsboro, NJ: Novo Nordisk; 2014
[23]Pi-Sunyer et al. [21]
[24]Davies et al. [22]
[25]Wadden et al. [23]

Phentermine/topiramate ER is a good choice for this patient. While phentermine monotherapy is also an option, the topiramate in phentermine/topiramate ER could also prevent her migraines, which occur frequently. Before prescribing the medication, confirm that the patient is not pregnant. The FDA requires a Risk Evaluation and Mitigation Strategy (REMS) so patients and prescribers are informed about the risk of orofacial clefts in infants exposed to topiramate during the first trimester of pregnancy [9]. The REMS addresses pregnancy prevention, consistent use of birth control, and importance of discontinuing phentermine/topiramate ER if pregnancy occurs.

In addition to anxiety or history of nephrolithiasis, make sure the patient does not have other contraindications including active or unstable coronary disease, hyperthyroidism, glaucoma, insomnia, or history of drug abuse of recent monoamine oxidase inhibitor use. The most common adverse events (AEs) reported in phase III trials were paresthesia, dry mouth, and constipation [10–12].

Orlistat is not an appropriate option for this patient because of her IBS-D. The gastrointestinal AEs including fecal urgency, oily stool, and fecal incontinence are difficult for many patients to tolerate [13]. As a result, orlistat is not commonly used for weight management. One exception is patients who are constipated and desire weight loss. The addition of a fiber supplement and slow dose titration can reduce AEs.

Lorcaserin is also not a good option for this patient because she is on high-dose sertraline. There is a theoretical interaction between lorcaserin and other serotonergic agents as coadministration may lead to serotonin syndrome or neuroleptic malignant syndrome-like reactions. Additionally, there is a theoretic risk of cardiac valvulopathy. Fenfluramine, a 5-HT2B-receptor agonist, was withdrawn from the market for this reason. Lorcaserin, however, binds selectively to the 5-HT2C receptors, and increased incidence of cardiac valvulopathy was not reported in the phase III trials [14, 15]. The most commonly reported AE is headache [14–16].

Naltrexone SR/bupropion SR could be an appropriate choice for this patient as there are no contraindications (including opioid use or history of seizure); however, phentermine/topiramate ER is a better option given her frequent migraines. If she does not tolerate the phentermine/topiramate ER or if it is not effective, other agents – including naltrexone SR/bupropion SR – should certainly be tried. Naltrexone SR/bupropion SR is a particularly good choice for patients who describe cravings and addictive food behavior as the phase III trials reported reduced frequency of food cravings, reduced difficulty resisting food cravings, and increased ability to control eating among patients taking the medication [17, 18]. The most commonly reported AEs in phase III trials were nausea, constipation, and headache [17–20].

Finally, liraglutide 3.0 mg could also be an appropriate choice for this patient as there are no contraindications, but she might not want to start with an injectable medication when there are oral alternatives. Liraglutide 3.0 mg can be an attractive option for patients who have anxiety or another condition that prevents use of stimulating medications. The most common adverse events (AEs) reported in phase III trials were nausea, constipation, and diarrhea [21–23].

Management

The patient was started on phentermine/topiramate ER 3.75/23 mg daily, which is the starting dose, and she was instructed to increase to 7.5/46 mg daily after 14 days. Counseling on dietary interventions and physical activity was provided. She had appointments with a registered dietitian after 4 and 8 weeks. She returned for a follow-up appointment at 12 weeks and was found to have lost 14 lbs (7% of her total body weight). As her weight loss was ongoing (she had not yet reached a plateau) and she did not describe increased hunger or cravings (symptoms of metabolic adaptation), the same dose of phentermine/topiramate ER was continued. According to manufacturer's instructions, if 3% weight loss is not achieved after 12 weeks on phentermine/topiramate ER, the medication should be discontinued, or the dose should be escalated. For escalation, a titration dose of 11.25/69 mg is taken daily for 2 weeks and then increased to a maintenance dose of 15/92 mg daily. The medication should be discontinued if 5% weight loss is not achieved after 12 weeks on 15/92 mg daily.

Outcome

Over the next few months, the patient's weight loss slowed down, and she reached a weight plateau so the dose of phentermine/topiramate ER was increased gradually to 15/92 mg daily. At this dose, she started to lose weight again and stopped suffering from migraines, and her lipid profile improved significantly. She continues to follow up with her providers at least once every 3 months to reinforce behavioral interventions and assess efficacy and safety of phentermine/topiramate ER.

Clinical Pearls and Pitfalls

- Patients who are obese or overweight with cardiovascular risk factors should be counseled on diet, physical activity, and other lifestyle modifications; however, weight loss achieved by behavioral changes alone is often limited and difficult to maintain [2–4].
- Anti-obesity pharmacotherapy can be considered for patients who have a BMI $\geq$ 30 kg/m^2 or $\geq$ 27 kg/m^2 with weight-related comorbidities including type 2 diabetes, hypertension, dyslipidemia, and obstructive sleep apnea [1, 5].
- Before starting pharmacotherapy for obesity, it is important to ask two questions:

   1) Are there contraindications, drug-drug interactions, or undesirable adverse effects associated with this medication that could be problematic for the patient?
   2) Can this medication improve other symptoms or conditions the patient has?

- As obesity is a chronic disease, most of the anti-obesity agents are approved for long-term use. When an anti-obesity medication is discontinued, there may be some weight regain.
- Weight loss of 5–10% in patients who are obese or overweight can lead to a clinically significant reduction in cardiovascular disease risk [6, 7].

References

1. Jensen MD, Ryan DH, Apovian CM, et al. 2013 AHA/ACC/TOS guideline for the management of overweight and obesity in adults: a report of the American College of Cardiology/American Heart Association task force on practice guidelines and the Obesity Society. J Am Coll Cardiol. 2014;63(25 Pt B):2985–3023.
2. Fothergill E, Guo J, Howard L, et al. Persistent metabolic adaptation 6 years after "the biggest loser" competition. Obesity (Silver Spring). 2016;24:1612–9.
3. Greenway FL. Physiological adaptations to weight loss and factors favouring weight regain. Int J Obes. 2015;39:1188–96.
4. Sumithran P, Predergast LA, Delbridge E, et al. Long-term persistence of hormonal adaptations to weight loss. N Engl J Med. 2011;365:1597–604.
5. Apovian CM, Aronne LJ, Bessesen DH, et al. Pharmacological management of obesity: an endocrine society clinical practice guideline. J Clin Endocrinol Metab. 2015;100:342–62.
6. Magkos F, Fraterrigo G, Yoshino J. Effects of moderate and subsequent progressive weight loss on metabolic function and adipose tissue biology in humans with obesity. Cell Metab. 2016;23:591–601.
7. Wing RR, Lang W, Wadden TA, et al. Benefits of modest weight loss in improving cardiovascular risk factors in overweight and obese individuals with type 2 diabetes. Diabetes Care. 2011;34:1481–6.
8. Saunders KH, Shukla AP, Igel LI, Aronne LJ. Obesity: when to consider medication. J Fam Pract. 2017;66(10):608–16.
9. Qsymia Risk Evaluation and Mitigation Strategy (REMS). VIVUS, Inc. Available at: http://www.qsymiarems.com. Accessed 25 Nov 2017.

10. Allison DB, Gadde KM, Garvey WT, et al. Controlled-release phentermine/topiramate in severely obese adults: a randomized controlled trial (EQUIP). Obesity (Silver Spring). 2012;20(2):330–42.
11. Gadde KM, Allison DB, Ryan DH, et al. Effects of low-dose, controlled-release, phentermine plus topiramate combination on weight and associated comorbidities in overweight and obese adults (CONQUER): a randomized, placebo-controlled, phase 3 trial. Lancet. 2011;377(9774):1341–52.
12. Garvey WT, Ryan DH, Look M, et al. Two-year sustained weight loss and metabolic benefits with controlled-release phentermine/topiramate in obese and overweight adults (SEQUEL): a randomized, placebo-controlled, phase 3 extension study. Am J Clin Nutr. 2012;95:297–308.
13. Torgerson JS, Hauptman J, Boldrin MN, et al. XENical in the prevention of diabetes in obese subjects (XENDOS) study: a randomized study of orlistat as an adjunct to lifestyle changes for the prevention of type 2 diabetes in obese patients. Diabetes Care. 2004;27:155–61.
14. Smith SR, Weissman NJ, Anderson CM, et al. Multicenter, placebo-controlled trial of lorcaserin for weight management. N Engl J Med. 2010;363:245–56.
15. Fidler MC, Sanchez M, Raether B, et al. A one-year randomized trial of lorcaserin for weight loss in obese and overweight adults: the BLOSSOM trial. J Clin Endocrinol Metab. 2011;96(10):3067–77.
16. O'Neil PM, Smith SR, Weissman NJ, et al. Randomized placebo controlled clinical trial of lorcaserin for weight loss in type 2 diabetes mellitus: the BLOOM-DM study. Obesity (Silver Spring). 2012;20(7):1426–36.
17. Greenway FL, Fujioka K, Plodkowski RA, et al. Effect of naltrexone plus bupropion on weight loss in overweight and obese adults (COR-I): a multicentre, randomised, double-blind, placebo-controlled, phase 3 trial. Lancet. 2010;376:595–605.
18. Apovian CM, Aronne L, Rubino D, et al. A randomized, phase 3 trial of naltrexone SR/bupropion SR on weight and obesity-related risk factors (COR-II). Obesity (Silver Spring). 2013;21:935–43.
19. Wadden TA, Foreyt JP, Foster GD, et al. Weight loss with naltrexone SR/bupropion SR combination therapy as an adjunct to behavior modification: the COR-BMOD trial. Obesity (Silver Spring). 2011;19:110–20.

20. Hollander P, Gupta AK, Plodkowski R, et al. Effects of naltrexone sustained-release/bupropion sustained-release combination therapy on body weight and glycemic parameters in overweight and obese patients with type 2 diabetes. Diabetes Care. 2013;36:4022–9.
21. Pi-Sunyer X, Astrup A, Fujioka K, et al. A randomized, controlled trial of 3.0 mg of liraglutide in weight management. N Engl J Med. 2015;373:11–22.
22. Davies MJ, Bergenstal R, Bode B, et al. Efficacy of liraglutide for weight loss among patients with type 2 diabetes: the SCALE diabetes randomized clinical trial. JAMA. 2015;314:687–99.
23. Wadden TA, Hollander P, Klein S, et al. Weight maintenance and additional weight loss with liraglutide after low-calorie-diet induced weight loss: the SCALE maintenance randomized study. Int J Obes. 2013;37:1443–51.
24. Igel LI, Kumar RB, Saunders KH, et al. Practical use of pharmacotherapy for obesity. Gastroenterology. 2017;152:1765–177. pii: S0016–5085(17)30142–7.
25. Saunders KH, Kumar RB, Igel LI, Aronne LJ. Pharmacologic approaches to weight management: recent gains and shortfalls in combating obesity. Curr Atheroscler Rep. 2016;18(7):36.
26. Aronne LJ, Wadden TA, Peterson C, Winslow D, Odeh S, Gadde KM. Evaluation of phentermine and topiramate versus phentermine/topiramate extended-release in obese adults. Obesity (Silver Spring). 2013;21(11):2163–71.

Chapter 14
Anti-Obesity Pharmacotherapy After Bariatric Surgery

Katherine H. Saunders

Case Presentation

A 63-year-old man is referred from his bariatric surgeon to an obesity medicine specialist for weight management. Four years ago, he underwent Roux-en-Y gastric bypass and lost 129 lbs or 38% of his total body weight (BMI 48.5 kg/m^2, 348 lbs, 5′11″ → BMI 30.5 kg/m^2, 219 lbs). He maintained this weight for 2 years; however, he has since regained 27 lbs (BMI 30.5 kg/m^2, 219 lbs → BMI 34.3 kg/m^2, 246 lbs). In addition to obesity, he suffers from type 2 diabetes, congestive heart failure, coronary artery disease, and hyperlipidemia. A recent transthoracic echocardiogram revealed normal valvular function. Following bariatric surgery, his hemoglobin A1c (HbA1c) improved, and he was able to discontinue all of his antidiabetic medications; however, his HbA1c increased to 7.9% last year, so metformin was restarted and titrated up to 1000 mg twice daily. His other medications are aspirin

K. H. Saunders (✉)
Comprehensive Weight Control Center, Division of Endocrinology, Diabetes and Metabolism, Weill Cornell Medical College, New York, NY, USA
e-mail: kph2001@med.cornell.edu

L. J. Aronne, R. B. Kumar (eds.), *Obesity Management*,
https://doi.org/10.1007/978-3-030-01039-3_14

81 mg daily, carvedilol 25 mg twice daily, lisinopril 10 mg daily, and rosuvastatin 10 mg daily. He follows a low-carbohydrate diet and exercises for 60 min most days of the week. He is concerned about his increasing weight and blood sugar. He denies pancreatitis and a personal or family history of medullary thyroid carcinoma. His exam is within normal limits, and his laboratory data reveal no abnormalities besides HbA1c of 7.4%. A few months ago, his primary care doctor initiated lorcaserin 10 mg twice daily for weight management. After 12 weeks, he had not lost any weight so the medication was discontinued.

Assessment and Diagnosis

This patient initially had class III obesity (BMI ≥ 40 kg/m^2) treated with bariatric surgery. He currently presents with class I obesity (BMI 30–34.9 kg/m^2) complicated by type 2 diabetes, congestive heart failure, coronary artery disease, and hyperlipidemia. As he has failed lifestyle modifications and a trial of lorcaserin, he is a good candidate for another anti-obesity agent in addition to ongoing lifestyle interventions.

Lorcaserin was an appropriate medication for the patient's internist to prescribe as there were no contraindications. In addition, the medication is associated with improved glycemic control. The BLOOM-DM trial reported a mean reduction in HbA1c of 0.9% in the treatment group compared with a 0.4% reduction in the placebo group [1]. Interestingly, some patients do not respond to lorcaserin. The most likely explanation for this interpatient variability is that there are many causes of obesity and only some respond to the activation of the 5-HT2C pathway. As a result, the medication should be discontinued if the patient has not achieved at least 5% weight loss after 12 weeks. As short-term results predict long-term success, the other anti-obesity medications approved for long-term use also have stopping rules (Table 14.1).

Phentermine and phentermine/topiramate ER are not appropriate medications for this patient because of his heart disease. Naltrexone SR/bupropion SR and orlistat could be considered, but liraglutide 3.0 mg is the best option given his need for further glucose control. Before starting liraglutide 3.0 mg, patients should be asked about their history of pancreatitis given the possible increased risk. In addition, liraglutide is contraindicated in patients with a personal or family history of multiple endocrine neoplasia syndrome type 2 or medullary thyroid carcinoma. Although thyroid C-cell tumors have been described in rodents given supratherapeutic doses of liraglutide, there is no evidence of liraglutide causing C-cell tumors in humans [2]. Finally, blood sugar should be monitored closely in patients on insulin or insulin secretagogues as concomitant use of liraglutide can increase the risk of hypoglycemia.

The potential reduction in cardiovascular risk is another benefit of liraglutide 3.0 mg for this patient. The LEADER trial reported a significant mortality benefit with liraglutide 1.8 mg daily among patients with type 2 diabetes and high

TABLE 14.1 Stopping rules for anti-obesity medications approved for long-term use

Medication	**Discontinue if the patient has not lost…**
Orlistat	Not specified
Phentermine/topiramate extended release (ER)	≥3% body weight after 12 weeks on 7.5/46 mg daily (*or* increase dose at this point) ≥5% body weight after 12 weeks on 15/92 mg daily
Lorcaserin	≥5% body weight after 12 weeks
Naltrexone sustained release (SR)/bupropion SR	≥5% body weight after 12 weeks at the maintenance dose (16 weeks total)
Liraglutide 3.0 mg	≥4% body weight after 16 weeks

cardiovascular risk. The study found that the rate of the first occurrence of death from cardiovascular causes, nonfatal myocardial infarction, or nonfatal stroke among patients with type 2 diabetes was lower with liraglutide than with placebo.

As weight regain following bariatric surgery is common, the use of anti-obesity medications can be an effective way to counteract recidivism and enhance weight maintenance [3]. Although there is limited data, the ideal time to begin an anti-obesity agent appears to be when patients reach a nadir weight rather than after weight regain has occurred [3]. In addition to pharmacotherapy following surgery, anti-obesity agents can be prescribed before bariatric procedures as well. The combination of medications with bariatric surgery (as well as endoscopic metabolic therapies and weight loss devices) is the areas that require further investigation.

Finally, many patients require more than one medication to achieve and maintain clinically significant weight loss. Combination therapy can have an additive or synergistic effect on weight by targeting multiple pathways simultaneously. In addition to naltrexone SR/bupropion SR and phentermine/topiramate ER, other combinations of agents are under investigation. An alternative to initiating two medications simultaneously is a stepwise approach in which an additional agent is added when a patient reaches a weight plateau. The combination of anti-obesity medications also requires further investigation.

Management

The patient was started on liraglutide 0.6 mg daily for 1 week with instructions to increase by 0.6 mg weekly to a therapeutic dosage of 3.0 mg daily. After 1 week, the patient called to report nausea with his first dose of liraglutide 1.2 mg daily. As a result, a slower dose titration was advised to reduce gastrointestinal side effects. (*Note*: this dose titration schedule does not follow manufacturer's guidelines, so it is technically off-label use.) Another option would have been an SGLT-2 inhibitor to treatment diabetes and facilitate weight loss.

He met with a registered dietitian monthly who provided ongoing dietary and exercise counseling. At his 16-week follow-up appointment, he was found to have lost 11 lbs (4.5% of his total body weight). As his weight loss had stopped (he had reached a plateau), the dose of liraglutide was increased from 1.2 to 1.8 mg daily at this visit. Again, a slow dose titration was advised to prevent side effects. The medication did not need to be discontinued according to manufacturer's instructions since the patient had lost at least 4% of his total body weight at 16 weeks.

Outcome

Over the next few months, the patient continued to lose weight and reduce his HbA1c to 6.8%. He continues to follow up with his providers at least once every 3 months to reinforce behavioral interventions and assess the efficacy and safety of liraglutide 3.0 mg daily.

Clinical Pearls and Pitfalls

- If feasible, assess efficacy and safety at least monthly for the first 3 months and then at least every 3 months in all patients prescribed anti-obesity pharmacotherapy [4].
- If a patient's response to an anti-obesity agent is deemed effective (weight loss ≥5% of body weight at 3 months or according to the manufacturers' individual stopping rules – Table 14.1) and safe, continue the medication. If deemed ineffective or if there are safety or tolerability issues at any time, discontinue the medication, and consider alternative medications or referral for an alternative treatment approach [4].
- Anti-obesity pharmacotherapy can be an effective tool to counteract recidivism and enhance weight maintenance after bariatric surgery, but this is an area that requires further investigation.

- Many patients require more than one medication to achieve and maintain clinically significant weight loss, and combination therapy can have an additive or synergistic effect on weight; however, this is also an area that requires further investigation.

References

1. O'Neil PM, Smith SR, Weissman NJ, et al. Randomized placebo controlled clinical trial of lorcaserin for weight loss in type 2 diabetes mellitus: the BLOOM-DM study. Obesity (Silver Spring). 2012;20:1426–36.
2. Madsen LW, Knauf JA, Gotfredsen C, et al. GLP-1 receptor agonists and the thyroid: C-cell effects in mice are mediated via the GLP-1 receptor and not associated with RET activation. Endocrinology. 2012;153(3):1538–47.
3. Stanford FC, Alfaris N, Gomez G, et al. The utility of weight loss medications after bariatric surgery for weight regain or inadequate weight loss: a multi-center study. Surg Obes Relat Dis. 2017;13(3):491–500.
4. Apovian CM, Aronne LJ, Bessesen DH, et al. Pharmacological management of obesity: an endocrine society clinical practice guideline. J Clin Endocrinol Metab. 2015;100:342–62.

Part VIII
Genetic Syndromes with Obesity

Chapter 15
Melanocortin 4 Receptor (MC4R) Deficiency

Ana B. Emiliano

Case Presentation

An 18-year-old female student comes for an evaluation, accompanied by her parents. She has been considering bariatric surgery to manage her long-standing history of obesity. The patient reports that since early childhood, she has had "weight issues." Her parents remember that at 12 months of age, she was always hungry and constantly seeking food. She was overweight as a toddler, but because of a history of overweight in her first paternal cousins, her parents did not think much of it. The patient's family has a very active lifestyle, which involves outdoor sports and hiking, so from an early age, she has been physically active. She currently plays lacrosse and field hockey at school, in addition to running 5 miles daily with her father. Her siblings – one brother and a sister – are lean, as well as the patient's mother. Her father is slightly overweight, in spite of his high activity level, and he was obese as a child. The patient feels that the most difficult part of trying to lose weight is controlling her appetite. She

A. B. Emiliano (✉)
The Rockefeller University, Clinician at the Comprehensive Weight Control Center, Weill Cornell Medical Center, New York, NY, USA
e-mail: aemiliano@rockefeller.edu

L. J. Aronne, R. B. Kumar (eds.), *Obesity Management*,
https://doi.org/10.1007/978-3-030-01039-3_15

has food thoughts most of the time, and it is hard to stay on a low-carbohydrate diet. She is frustrated that no matter how much she exercises, she does not seem able to lose weight. At the moment, she weighs 120 kg, and her height is 1.80 m. The patient is much taller than her mother and siblings and as tall as her father. She currently takes no medications. Menarche was at age 13 and her menses are regular. She is doing well academically but feels her social life is restricted by her feeling ashamed of her weight. On her physical exam, her vital signs were within normal range. The patient looked her stated age. The exam revealed central adiposity but no dysmorphic features or acanthosis nigricans.

Assessment and Diagnosis

The most prevalent form of obesity is known as "common" obesity. It results from a combination of genetic predisposition and environmental factors, including diet, physical activity, and socioeconomic status, among others. The genetic predisposition to obesity is reflected in the heritability of BMI, which has been estimated at 40–70%, based on the data from twin and adoption studies [1, 2]. More than 200 loci have been linked to common obesity in genome-wide association studies (GWAS), representing genetic variability in the general population associated with a high BMI [3, 4]. Common obesity results from the cumulative effects of multiple gene variants and, therefore, has been also deemed "polygenic" obesity. On the other hand, genetic obesity syndromes are rare forms of obesity, representing approximately 1% of all forms of adult obesity [5]. They arise from genetic defects (mutations/deletions/imprinting defects/translocation) involving a single gene or a group of genes on a given chromosomal segment [6]. Based on the number of genes involved and the presence or absence of developmental delay, genetic obesity syndromes are classified as either *non-syndromic monogenic obesity* or *syndromic obesity*. Non-syndromic monogenic obesity, as the name implies, can be traced to mutations of a single gene and does not involve pleiotropic manifestations, unlike syndromic obesity. The hallmark of non-syndromic monogenic obesity is severe hyperphagia and obesity (Table 15.1). Many of the genes involved in non-syndromic monogenic obesity are part of central leptin-melanocortin signaling pathways [7], underscoring the brain's fundamental role in regulating energy homeostasis.

Although pediatric obesity is becoming more prevalent, a history of early childhood obesity and excessive, unusual, food-seeking behaviors should prompt a clinician to consider a genetic obesity syndrome. In the case described above, the patient was reported to have developed hyperphagia early in childhood, and she was overweight as a toddler. While her intense physical activity may have curtailed more significant weight gain, the patient has moderate obesity, at a BMI of 37. The fact that her father has a history of childhood obesity, which is absent in her siblings' and mother's history, also suggests the possibility of a genetic obesity syndrome, given the pattern of segregation. Her paternal cousins also have a history of obesity, as well as her paternal uncle and grandmother. The absence of dysmorphic features, intellectual disabilities, and a history of normal puberty speak against syndromic obesity. The patient is taller than her siblings. Given that MC4R deficiency is the most common non-syndromic monogenic obesity and is associated with increased linear growth, it should be considered in the differential diagnosis.

Emerging therapies to treat non-syndromic monogenic forms of obesity increase the relevance of identifying such conditions in patients with obesity. In the past, only leptin deficiency was amenable to pharmacological treatment, with leptin replacement therapy. However, the development of the MC4R agonist setmelanotide has provided a therapy for POMC deficiency, and there is promise it may be helpful for leptin receptor deficiency, as well [8, 9]. At the time of the writing of this chapter, there were no available pharmacological treatments for the other forms of non-syndromic monogenic obesity, other than maintaining a low-calorie diet with regular physical activity and pharmacological treatment of

Table 15.1 Non-syndromic monogenic obesity

Non-syndromic monogenic obesity	Genetics	Prevalence	Manifestations
Leptin deficiency	Leptin gene; autosomal recessive	1% of severely obese individuals	Hyperphagia, hyperinsulinemia, early-onset childhood obesity, severe obesity
Leptin receptor deficiency	Leptin receptor gene; autosomal recessive	2–3% of severely obese individuals	Hyperphagia, hyperinsulinemia, hyperleptinemia, early-onset childhood obesity, severe obesity; spontaneous but delayed puberty
Pro-opiomelanocortin deficiency	POMC gene; recessive; individuals affected are homozygous or compound heterozygous	Rare	Newborns have secondary adrenal insufficiency; patients require corticosteroid replacement for life; pale skin; red hair in Caucasians; obesity
Prohormone Convertase 1	PCSK-1 gene; recessive; individuals affected are homozygous or compound heterozygous	Rare	Newborns have secondary adrenal insufficiency; early-onset childhood obesity; hypogonadotropic hypogonadism; postprandial hypoglycemia

Melanocortin 4 receptor deficiency	MC4R gene; codominant mode of expression; occasionally homozygous	5% of severely obese individuals	Early-onset hyperphagia; increased bone mineral density; increased linear growth during childhood; severity of obesity depends on environmental factors
Single-minded 1 deficiency	SIM1 gene; chromosomal rearrangements or heterozygous missense mutations; transcription factor involved in the development of paraventricular and supraoptic hypothalamic nuclei	Rare	Early-onset hyperphagia; severe obesity

diabetes and hyperlipidemia. Bariatric surgery can, sometimes, be helpful, as well as medications used to treat common types of obesity (see Chap. 14). When the medical history is suggestive of a genetic obesity syndrome, genetic testing is indicated. However, most patients with non-syndromic monogenic obesity present with obesity in early childhood, so it would be unusual for a patient to be diagnosed as an adult.

Management

The laboratory tests did not show evidence of abnormal glucose homeostasis or hyperlipidemia. A sleep study did not reveal sleep apnea. Given her BMI of 37 and the absence of comorbidities, the patient did not qualify for bariatric surgery. The initial recommendation was for the patient to work with a nutritionist and continue to exercise regularly, with a main focus on gaining muscle mass through strength training. At that time, however, the patient was already engaging in vigorous physical activity. Based on the medical history and presentation, genetic testing was recommended in a Clinical Laboratory Improvement Amendments (CLIA)-certified laboratory. A non-syndromic monogenic obesity sequencing panel including the exons and exon-intron junctions of the genes listed in Table 15.1 was ordered. The patient was found to be heterozygous for the P.Cys271Arg MC4R mutation, which results in loss of function of the MC4R gene [10]. Testing of her father also revealed the same MC4R mutation. Her siblings and mother tested negative. Relatives, including her paternal cousins and grandmother, refused testing.

MC4R is a seven-transmembrane G-coupled receptor found in the paraventricular hypothalamic nucleus. When activated by its ligand, alpha-melanocyte-stimulating hormone (α-MSH), MC4R promotes satiety, energy expenditure, and weight loss [11]. MC4R deficiency is the most common monogenic type of obesity, with a prevalence between 1 and 6% among severely obese individuals [12].

Heterozygous individuals for MC4R mutations can have variable phenotypes, ranging from mild overweight to severe obesity, depending on the type of mutation (inactive or partially inactive), penetrance, and environmental factors [6]. Penetrance of MC4R mutations is incomplete in heterozygous individuals, and hyperphagia and obesity are always more pronounced in individuals who are homozygous for MC4R mutations [13]. The mode of inheritance of MC4R deficiency is described as codominant, as the two alleles influence the phenotype [12]. The natural history of MC4R deficiency often courses with a decrease in the intensity of the hyperphagia, as individuals enter adulthood, with obesity becoming less severe [14].

The management of MC4R deficiency patients includes a low-calorie diet, exercise, general pharmacological therapies directed to manage obesity, and bariatric surgery. To date, there is no specific treatment for MC4R deficiency. If the patient met the inclusion criteria for bariatric surgery, that type of therapy should be considered. Durable weight loss has been achieved in patients with MC4R deficiency that underwent bariatric surgery, although there is no consensus on whether it should be universally recommended [5, 10].

Outcome

The patient expressed frustration with not being able to lose any weight after 6 months of intense dieting, exercise, and a trial of metformin, followed by a GLP-1 agonist. In spite of working closely with her physician and dietitian, she only lost 4 pounds. After a discussion with her physician, in her parents' presence, considering the pros and cons of bariatric surgery, the patient and her family felt that bariatric surgery would be the best option for her. In the absence of effective treatment, the patient reached a BMI of 40, and was able to obtain health insurance coverage for bariatric surgery. The procedure selected was Roux-en-Y gastric bypass.

She underwent the surgery without complications. One year after the surgery, she had lost 30% total body weight and was still losing weight, but at a slower pace. Her BMI 1 year after the surgery was 26. She was extremely compliant with her diet and supplement therapy, which included a multivitamin containing 200% of the recommended dietary allowance for iron, folic acid, and thiamine, in addition to copper, selenium, and zinc. She also took daily vitamin B12, calcium citrate, and vitamin D [15].

The patient continued to be followed in the weight management clinic, alternating appointments with a nutritionist and physician every 4 months. In terms of genetic counseling, if the patient were to have children, there would be a 50% chance she would transmit the MC4R mutation to her offspring. The degree of penetrance and severity of the phenotype would depend on codominant factors and whether her male partner would also have MC4R deficiency. Since she would not consider having children until reaching her 30s, the patient prefers to defer these considerations to the future.

Clinical Pearls and Pitfalls

- A history of severe hyperphagia and childhood obesity should raise the suspicion for a genetic obesity syndrome.
- Non-syndromic monogenic obesity is characterized by hyperphagia and severe obesity, manifesting during childhood.
- MC4R deficiency is the most prevalent non-syndromic monogenic obesity form.
- Bariatric surgery can be a therapeutic option for individuals with MC4R deficiency, if other interventions prove unhelpful.
- Close monitoring by a physician specialized in obesity management and a nutritionist can help patients achieve and maintain healthier BMIs and prevent weight regain after bariatric surgery.

- Patients with non-syndromic monogenic obesity should also be closely monitored for the development of obesity comorbidities, including type 2 diabetes, hypertension, hyperlipidemia, heart disease, and sleep apnea, and should have their routine cancer screening up-to-date.

References

1. Barsh GS, Farooqi IS, O'Rahilly S. Genetics of body-weight regulation. Nature. 2000;404:644–51.
2. Allison DB, Kaprio J, Korkeila M, et al. The heritability of body mass index among an international sample of monozygotic twins reared apart. Int J Obes Relat Metab Disord. 1996;20:501–6.
3. Locke AE, Kahali B, Berndt SI, et al. Genetic studies of body mass index yield new insights for obesity biology. Nature. 2015;518:197–206.
4. Akiyama M, Okada Y, Kanai M, et al. Genome-wide association study identifies 112 new loci for body mass index in the Japanese population. Nat Genet. 2017;49:1458–67.
5. Farooqi IS, O'Rahilly S. The genetics of obesity in humans. In: De Groot LJ, Chrousos G, Dungan K, et al., editors. *Endotext* [Internet]. South Dartmouth: MDText.com, Inc.; 2017.
6. Chung WK. An overview of monogenic and syndromic obesities in humans. Pediatr Blood Cancer. 2012;58:122–8.
7. Zegers D, Van Hul W, Van Gaal LF, et al. Monogenic and complex forms of obesity: insights from genetics reveal the leptin-melanocortin signaling pathway as a common player. Crit Rev Eukaryot Gene Expr. 2012;22:325–43.
8. Clément K, Biebermann H, Farooqi IS, et al. MC4R agonism promotes durable weight loss in patients with leptin receptor deficiency. Nature Med. 2018. https://doi.org/10.1038/s41591-018-0015-9. [Epub ahead of print].
9. Kühnen P, Clément K, Wiegand S, et al. Proopiomelanocortin receptor deficiency treated with a melanocortin 4 receptor agonist. N Engl J Med. 2016;375:240–6.

10. Censani M, Conroy R, Deng L, et al. Weight loss after bariatric surgery in morbidly obese adolescents with *MC4R* mutations. Obesity (Silver Spring). 2014;22:225–31.
11. Krashes MJ, Lowell BB, Garfield AS. Melanocortin-4 receptor-regulated energy homeostasis. Nat Neurosci. 2016;19:206–19.
12. Farooqi IS, Yeo GS, Keogh JM, et al. Dominant and recessive inheritance of morbid obesity associated with melanocortin 4 receptor deficiency. J Clin Invest. 2000;106:271–9.
13. Stutzmann F, et al. Prevalence of melanocortin-4 receptor deficiency in Europeans and their age-dependent penetrance in multigenerational pedigrees. Diabetes. 2008;57:2511–8.
14. Lubrano-Berthelier C, Cavazos M, Dubern B, et al. Molecular genetics of human obesity – associated MC4R mutations. Ann N Y Acad Sci. 2003;994:49–57.
15. Kim TY, Kim S, Schafer AL. Medical Management of the Postoperative Bariatric Surgery Patient. In: De Groot LJ, Chrousos G, Dungan K, et al., editors. Endotext [Internet]. South Dartmouth: MDText.com, Inc.; 2018.

Chapter 16
Prader-Willi Syndrome (PWS)

Ana B. Emiliano

Case Presentation

A 23-year-old male with a history of Prader-Willi syndrome (PWS) comes for an initial visit for obesity management. His parents, who accompany him, report that the patient is now at his highest weight, after a failed attempt to live in a group home where his food intake was not being closely monitored. Three years ago, while living at home, he achieved his lowest adult weight, at 95 kg, through a rigorous regime including a low-calorie diet and physical activity, closely monitored by his parents. However, as the patient became increasingly aggressive and oppositional due to his uncontrollable hyperphagia and behavioral issues, his parents decided he should live in a group home. After 6 months in the group home, the patient reached his highest adult weight, at 130 kg, and developed prediabetes, with a hemoglobin A1c of 5.9%. His height is 1.70 m and his BMI is 45. He also has mild hypertension and sleep apnea. The patient now is back at home, living with his parents, and with the help of an aide, they have been able to

A. B. Emiliano (✉)
The Rockefeller University, Clinician at the Comprehensive Weight Control Center, Weill Cornell Medical Center, New York, NY, USA
e-mail: aemiliano@rockefeller.edu

L. J. Aronne, R. B. Kumar (eds.), *Obesity Management*,
https://doi.org/10.1007/978-3-030-01039-3_16

restrict his access to food. The patient is described as having an uncontrollable appetite, and if his parents and caretaker forget to lock the refrigerator and kitchen cabinets, the patient will eat all edibles in sight. He has been calmer on the current medications but still grows frustrated with being hungry "all the time." The patient also displays significant skin picking. In terms of his past medical history, he had hypotonia, feeding difficulties, and failure to thrive during infancy. He walked at 12 months and had normal verbal development. He rapidly gained weight after age 4 and was already obese by age 8. As a teenager, he started to display aggressive behaviors, growing defiant and at times physically threatening when told he could not eat. He developed more severe obesity after being started on antipsychotics and mood stabilizers for behavioral problems. Testing at age 17 revealed an IQ of 70. Surgical history includes orchidopexy at 18 months of age. His current medications include metformin, aripiprazole, fluoxetine, propranolol, and testosterone gel. His parents heard of other patients with PWS being treated with a GLP-1 agonist and would like to consider that option for their son. The patient is an only child.

Assessment and Diagnosis

Syndromic obesity, as opposed to non-syndromic monogenic obesity, has pleiotropic manifestations, encompassing intellectual disabilities, dysmorphic features, and developmental abnormalities, in addition to obesity [1, 2]. Syndromic obesity can be due to single-gene mutations or to genetic abnormalities involving multiple genes on a chromosome. PWS is a classic example of syndromic obesity (Table 16.1).

PWS arises from the lack of expression of paternally inherited genes on chromosome 15q11.2–q13 imprinting region due to deletions, imprinting defects, maternal uniparental disomy, or paternal translocation errors [3]. Some of the genes affected include SNURF, SNORD116, SNRPN, MKRN3, and MAGEL 23. Neonatal hypotonia, feeding dif-

TABLE 16.1 Syndromic obesity

Syndromic obesity	Genetics	Prevalence	Manifestations
Prader-Willi syndrome	Lack of expression of a group of genes on paternal copy of chromosome 15q11.2–q13 imprinting region due to deletion, imprinting errors, or maternal uniparental disomy	1:10,000–30,000 births	Neonatal hypotonia, feeding difficulties, failure to thrive, dysmorphic features, developmental disabilities; hyperphagia and obesity developing in childhood and persisting into adulthood; behavioral and psychiatric disorders; skin picking
Bardet-Biedl syndrome	Autosomal recessive; >20 genes to date associated with the syndrome; defined as a ciliopathy	1:13,500–160,000 births	Intellectual disabilities, postaxial polydactyly, retinal dystrophy that can progress to legal blindness in adulthood, hypogonadism, renal disease, obesity, psychiatric disorders
Albright hereditary osteodystrophy	Autosomal dominant; maternally transmitted; mutations of GNAS1, leading to impaired function of Gsα protein	0.79:100,000 births	Pseudohypoparathyroidism type Ia: obesity; intellectual disabilities; PTH, TSH, GnRH, and GHRH resistance of variable degrees; skeletal abnormalities, including brachydactyly

(continued)

Table 16.1 (continued)

Syndromic obesity	Genetics	Prevalence	Manifestations
Alström syndrome	Autosomal recessive; homozygous or compound heterozygous mutations in the Alström syndrome protein 1; defined as a ciliopathy	1–9:1,000,000 births	Retinal dystrophy; renal disease; male hypogonadism; female hyperandrogenism; short stature; cardiomyopathy; hearing impairment; obesity
Wilms tumor, aniridia, genitourinary malformations, mental retardation (WAGR) syndrome	Autosomal dominant; de novo heterozygous deletion on chromosome 11p13, leading to haploinsufficiency of Wilms tumor 1 (WT1) and paired box 6 (PAX6) genes; when affecting the BDNF gene, resulting phenotype also includes obesity	1:1,000,000 births	Wilms tumor; aniridia; genitourinary malformations; intellectual disability; hyperphagia and obesity; genitourinary malformations
16p11.2 deletions or microdeletions	Autosomal dominant; copy number variant (deletions or microdeletions associated with obese phenotype); de novo event or inherited	Rare	Neuropsychiatric disorders; developmental delay; early-onset obesity

ficulties, and failure to thrive are very suggestive of PWS. The dysmorphic features associated with PWS include a narrow face, almond-shaped eyes, and a thin upper lip with down-turned mouth corners. Individuals with PWS usually have small hands and short stature. Intellectual disabilities and neuropsychiatric disorders are also characteristic, with oppositional defiant and aggressive behaviors. Hypogonadism is common, as well as defects in growth hormone (GH) secretion [4].

Clinical criteria developed in 1993 are still in use given its diagnostic accuracy [5]. Genetic testing is used to establish the diagnosis. The definitive test is methylation analysis, although fluorescence in situ hybridization (FISH) and chromosomal microarray are also utilized in the diagnosis of PWS [3].

In terms of genetic counseling, the risk of having other children with PWS depends on the disease mechanism. The probability is less than 1% when the paternal genes are not expressed due to a deletion or due to maternal uniparental disomy, up to 50% if secondary to an imprinting defect and up to 25% if due to chromosome translocation [3].

Management

The patient's family understands that the basic tenets of PWS management are restriction of access to food and increased physical activity, with firm limit setting. A low-carbohydrate diet and low-calorie diet at 1800 kcal/day, under the supervision of a nutritionist, would be recommended. In addition, regular physical exercise, consisting of at least 30 min of cardio daily and strength training approximately 3 times a week, should also be included. Because the patient is still gaining weight, it is important to review his medication list to assess if any of his medications may be exacerbating the PWS hyperphagia or preventing energy expenditure. Of his current medications, propranolol is the most likely to be preventing weight loss (see Chap. 7). Therefore, it would be helpful to discontinue propranolol and replace it with an antihypertensive that will not prevent weight loss, such as an ACE inhibitor. While metformin is a good choice for weight loss and prediabetes management, the patient may benefit from additional pharmacotherapy to prevent or stall progression to type 2 diabetes. A GLP-1 agonist, such as liraglutide, could be added to his regimen [6]. Topiramate would also be a good choice, as in addition to suppressing appetite, it may also decrease skin picking [6]. One important consideration for this patient would be assessing his plasma IGF-1 level, as patients with PWS often have growth hormone deficiency. If low, provocative testing should be performed under the supervision of an endocrinologist, in a licensed site, with either an insulin tolerance test or arginine-GHRH (growth hormone-releasing hormone) [7]. GH replacement may increase the patient's lean body mass and improve metabolism [6]. Therefore, working closely with an endocrinologist is advisable. Bariatric surgery may be helpful in PWS if patients are closely monitored and supervised [8].

Outcome

The patient was kept on a strict low-carbohydrate and low-calorie diet, in addition to daily physical activity. He was closely managed by his physician and nutritionist at the weight management clinic. Liraglutide, initially at 0.3 mg/day, was added to metformin and slowly increased to 1.2 mg, according to the patient's tolerance. An ACE inhibitor was substituted for propranolol. The patient was maintained on aripiprazole and fluoxetine, as his behavioral problems were under good control. After 6 months following these medication adjustments, the patient lost almost 11 kg but his weight loss plateaued at that level. Topiramate was added to help with the hyperphagia and skin picking, starting with 25 mg twice daily. The patient responded well to that addition, continuing to lose approximately 1 pound every other week in the subsequent months as the topiramate dose was titrated up. The patient also had two low plasma IGF-1 levels, on two separate occasions, at 84 mg/dl. A provocative GH test, with an insulin tolerance test, confirmed the diagnosis of GH deficiency. The patient was then started on GH replacement. Compliance with CPAP was increased with parental supervision.

Clinical Pearls and Pitfalls

- Syndromic obesity has pleiotropic manifestations, unlike non-syndromic monogenic obesity.
- PWS is the most common form of syndromic obesity.
- Although there is no specific treatment for PWS, a combination of diet, exercise, and behavioral and pharmacological interventions may lead to weight loss.
- Bariatric surgery may also be helpful but more research is needed.

References

1. Geets E, Meuwissen MEC, Van Hul W. Clinical, molecular genetics and therapeutic aspects of syndromic obesity. Clin Genet. 2018; https://doi.org/10.1111/cge.13367. [Epub ahead of print].
2. Mantovani G. Pseudohypoparathyroidism: diagnosis and treatment. J Clin Endocrinol Metab. 2011;96:3020–30.
3. Driscoll DJ, Miller JL, Schwartz S, et al. Prader-Willi syndrome. 1998 Oct 6 [Updated 2017 Dec 14]. In: Adam MP, Ardinger HH, Pagon RA, et al., editors. GeneReviews [Internet]. Seattle (WA): University of Washington; 1993–2018.
4. Angulo MA, Butler MG, Cataletto ME. Prader-Willi syndrome: a review of clinical, genetic, and endocrine findings. J Endocrinol Investig. 2015;38:1249–63.
5. Holm VA, et al. Prader-Willi syndrome: consensus diagnostic criteria. Pediatrics. 1993;91:398–402.
6. Goldstone AP, Holland AJ, Hauffa BP, Hokken-Koelega AC, Tauber M. On behalf of speakers and contributors at the second expert meeting of the Comprehensive Care of Patients with

PWS. Recommendations for the diagnosis and treatment of Prader Willi syndrome. J Clin Endocrinol Metab. 2008;93:4183–97.

7. Molitch ME, Clemmons DR, Malozowski S, Merriam GR, Vance ML. Evaluation and treatment of adult growth hormone deficiency: an Endocrine Society clinical practice guideline. J Clin Endocrinol Metab. 2011;96:1587–609.
8. Irizarry KA, Miller M, Freemark M, Haqq AM. Prader Willi syndrome: genetics, metabolomics, hormonal function, and new approaches to therapy. Adv Pediatr Infect Dis. 2016;63(1):47–77.

Index

L. J. Aronne, R. B. Kumar (eds.), *Obesity Management*,
https://doi.org/10.1007/978-3-030-01039-3

9783030010386